THE Age Well Plan

THE Age Well Plan

ACHIEVE HEALTH AND VITALITY AT ANY AGE

Edited by
EMMA VAN HINSBERGH

SIRIUS

SIRIUS

This edition published in 2023 by Sirius Publishing, a division of
Arcturus Publishing Limited,
26/27 Bickels Yard, 151–153 Bermondsey Street,
London SE1 3HA

ISBN: 978-1-3988-2042-5
AD008849UK

Printed in China

CONTENTS

6
INTRODUCTION

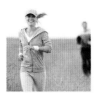

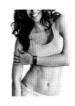

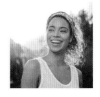

8
WHAT'S AGEING YOU?
Find out what may be causing you to age faster – and what you can do about it.

20
YOUR BODY
Learn how your body changes as you age, including hormones and digestion, bones and muscles.

40
YOUR MIND
High stress can be ageing, as can getting stuck in a rut. Here's how to keep your mind in the best shape.

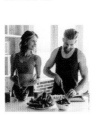

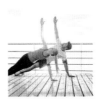

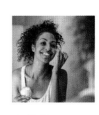

58
YOUR DIET
Some foods are particularly great for combating the ageing process – you can learn about them here.

84
YOUR FITNESS
Exercises that boost your heart, combined with strength training are the best way to general fitness.

102
YOUR FACE
While your face is a picture of your life, here's how to get and keep a glowing complexion.

INTRODUCTION

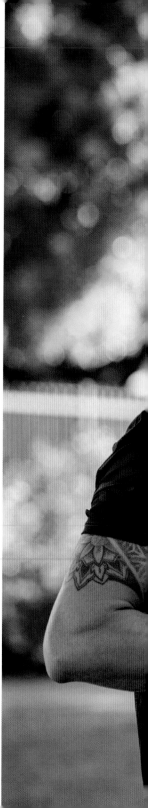

It's easy to associate ageing with fine lines and the odd grey hair and forget the positive benefits of being older – things that concerned you in your youth seem less important as you become more confident in yourself. And with each decade, new challenges and the skills you develop to meet them all go towards making you who you are.

So rather than thinking of age-proofing your body as a self-improvement regime, see it as looking after yourself as you age. It won't just make you look and feel younger and boost your health, it can be fun too! Of course, there's no magic pill, but taking a proactive approach to your health and wellbeing during each stage of your life will ensure you look and feel your best, whatever your age. So whether you're in your 20s, 30s, 40s or beyond, this book will give you all the age-specific tips you need to see the changes you want.

There are plenty of effective, natural steps you can take every day to stay looking and feeling younger. Scientific research is increasingly proving that your genetic make-up is not the only determinant of how quickly – or slowly – you age. Your diet, exercise, lifestyle habits and skincare regime all play a key role in how youthful you look and feel. The way you eat, breathe, sleep and even think can accelerate or slow down the ageing process.

This book shows you the latest, natural ways to turn back the clock. You'll find everything from anti-ageing skincare secrets to stay-young foods and the best exercises to keep you toned, strong and flexible.

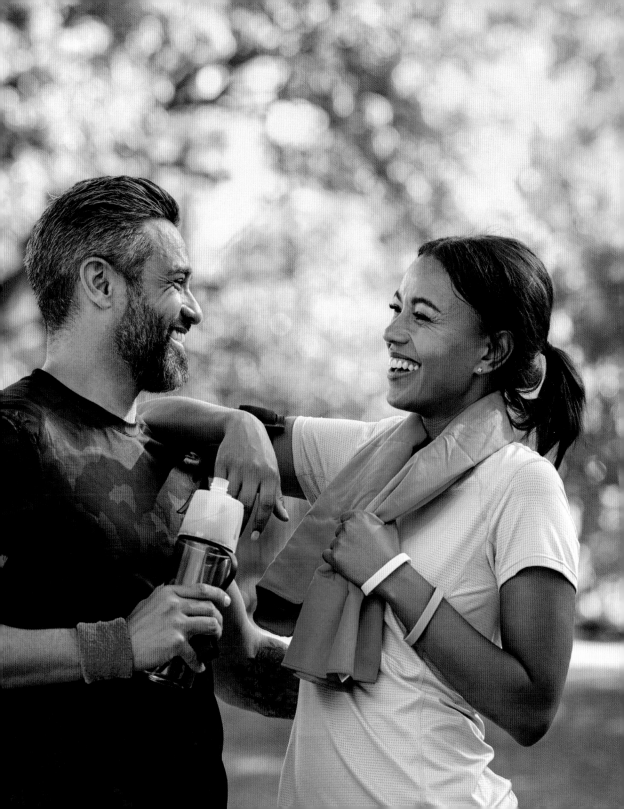

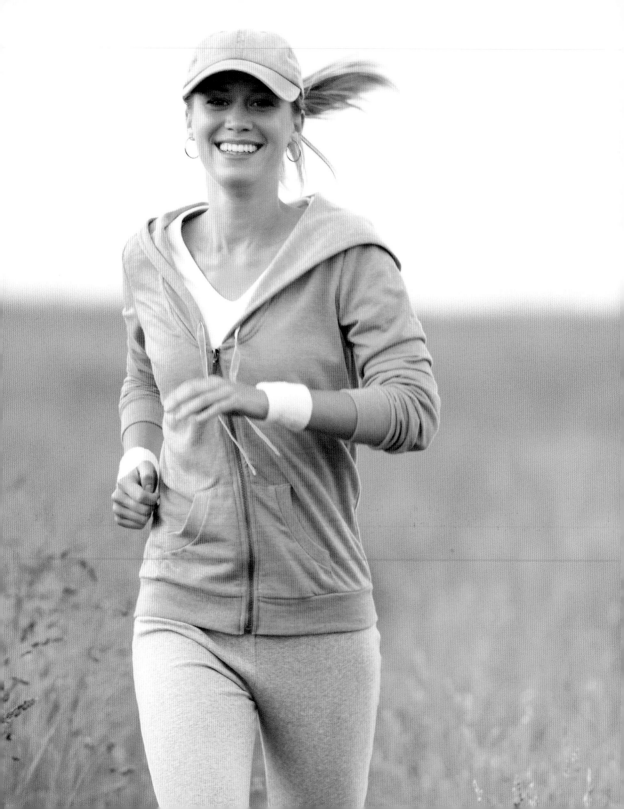

WHAT'S AGEING YOU?

Research shows that we have a great deal of control over our ageing process. We don't purely 'inherit' longevity; it's the sum total of our lifestyle habits. Learning how to make simple lifestyle changes – such as regular exercise, low alcohol intake and not smoking – can actually add as much as 14 extra years to your life!

AGE-RELATED FACTORS

Whether or not you look older or younger than your calendar age doesn't just depend on your genes. A cocktail of factors determine how fast you age.

The physical signs of ageing may be inevitable, but the pace at which they occur isn't. It's down to a mix of biological 'intrinsic' programming and external or 'extrinsic' factors. Here are the main age-related accelerators that are worth thinking about.

SEDENTARY LIFESTYLE

Exercise, or rather a lack of it, is one of the most powerful factors contributing to ageing — internally and externally. Staying active helps prevent many conditions and illnesses associated with old age, including heart disease, dementia and osteoporosis. It keeps you mobile for longer and, by boosting your circulation, makes your skin radiant. But, crucially, exercise also works at a cellular level and, as a result, strengthens your skeleton, improves your digestion and enlarges your heart. A study at King's College, London, and the National Institute on Ageing, Maryland in the US, found a couch-potato lifestyle can biologically age you by up to 10 years by shortening chain-like structures called telomeres, which work to protect DNA.

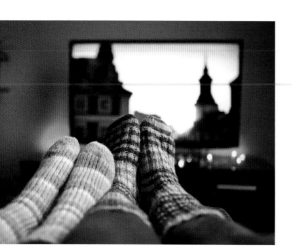

POOR DIET

Eating healthily is crucial for maintaining a healthy weight and preventing age-related diseases, and research shows it will also keep your skin looking youthful too. Choosing the right kind of foods — namely antioxidant-rich fruit and vegetables — can counteract the ageing effects of pesky free radicals. Drinking

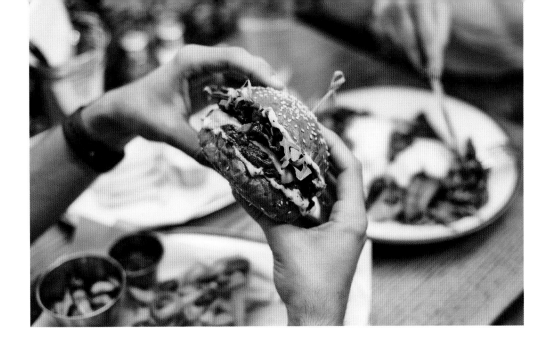

plenty of water and eating healthy fats, such as plant oils, are essential for keeping your complexion hydrated and plump.

In contrast, an excess of sugary, processed foods can accelerate the breakdown of collagen and elastin fibres, which act as your skin's scaffolding. Eating too much saturated animal fat can overburden your heart and liver, resulting in a dull and lifeless complexion.

SMOKING

There's no part of your body that isn't affected by smoking. It's detrimental to skin; not only does it decrease oxygen supply so your complexion appears dull and dehydrated, it also generates free radicals and causes those characteristic 'inhale' wrinkles around the mouth. It's said that regular smokers will eventually look 10 to 20 years older than their natural age, and no area of skin is left unsullied, according to experts at the University of Michigan in the US. Inside your body, smoking interferes with the renewal of bones, reducing their density, contributes to the furring of the arteries – a process called atherosclerosis – damages your lungs and significantly increases the likelihood of oral health problems, such as tooth loss.

SUN

In many ways a blast of sunshine is positively life-enhancing; it flushes your body with vitamin D, which is vital for a healthy immune system, balanced mood and strong bones. And, of course, aesthetically, sun-kissed skin has a natural, healthy glow. However, too much can be a bad thing. As well as increasing your risk of skin cancer, sun exposure is recognized as one of most potent complexion-agers, causing, according to dermatologists, a whopping 80 per cent of age-related skin damage. It can contribute to age spots, wrinkles, pigmentation and loss of elasticity. Plus, it ages your hair and eyes.

STRESS

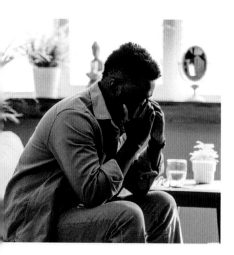

Stress used to be merely seen as a state of mind. But now, there's increasing evidence that chronic and prolonged episodes can compromise your health and age your body. Research shows it can disrupt sleep, dampen your immune system, contribute to raised blood pressure, and result in weight gain – which are all ageing. And don't forget that it can also directly contribute to the physical signs of ageing; all that frowning can lead to permanent lines on your forehead! Researchers at Case Western Reserve University in Cleveland, Ohio in the US who studied identical twins, who should age at a similar rate, found that a divorced twin looked almost two years older than their sibling who was single or married. The scientists suggested it was the sustained periods of stress that the divorced twins had been through that was one of the biggest factors in how much faster they aged. Your hair can suffer too – anxiety can thin and accelerate the greying process.

ALCOHOL

An occasional tipple won't do you any harm – in fact various studies, including a recent one on heart disease published in the *British Medical Journal*, show that moderate drinking is beneficial. However,

What are they?

Free radicals are atoms or groups of atoms in our bodies that have electrons missing, so they become highly chemically reactive. To redress their electron imbalance, these scavengers 'steal' electrons from other molecules in your body and, by altering their chemical structure, cause damage to cells, protein and DNA. This can result in increased signs of ageing, as well as contribute to degenerative diseases, such as cancer.

What triggers them?

Free radicals are created in response to your body's interaction with oxygen, and are caused by natural biological processes such as breathing, as well as external pollutants such as toxins and tobacco smoke.

How to combat them

To prevent cellular damage (oxidative stress), it's a good idea to increase your intake of antioxidants. Available in fresh fruit and vegetables, antioxidants mop up and neutralize dangerous free radicals and are central to your anti-ageing armour.

excess long-term consumption contributes to liver disease, heart problems, weakened bones and has been highlighted as a risk factor in breast cancer. And it's bad for your skin too. Alcohol can dehydrate your complexion, damage elastin and collagen, cause sensitivity and result in broken veins and a ruddy hue.

POLLUTION

On a day-to-day basis, we're bombarded by an array of polluting particles in our environment, from paint fumes to chemical air fresheners to the ultra-fine dust from photocopiers and toxic exhaust emissions from cars. Our lungs are, without doubt, affected — but so, too, is our skin. According to a recent study conducted at Leibniz Research Institute for Environmental Medicine in Dusseldorf in Germany, the higher the concentration of traffic-related airborne particles, the greater the likelihood of extrinsic skin ageing, particularly pigment spots on the forehead and cheeks.

WHAT'S YOUR REAL AGE?

Take this quiz to find out whether your chronological age matches up with your body.

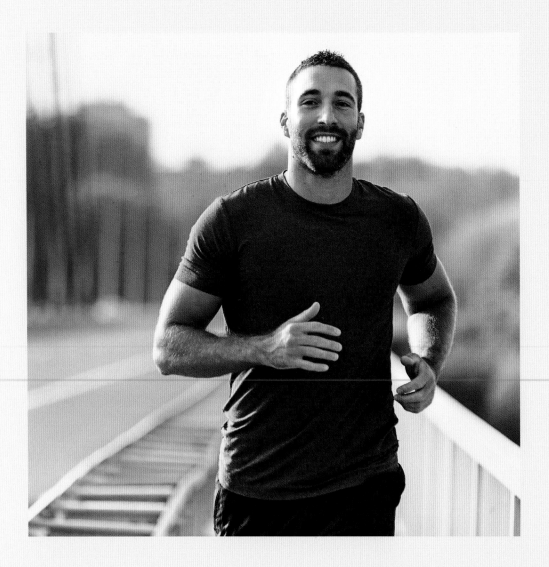

This quiz will help highlight the factors that may be prematurely ageing you. For each question, use the following scoring system, unless stated:

Yes, always – 1 point
Sometimes – 0.5 point
Frankly, no – 0 point

1. Research shows exercise is good for your heart, bones and brain, and reduces the risk of chronic illnesses. Aerobic exercise, such as swimming, walking and cycling, keeps your heart and lungs youthful. *Do you exercise aerobically every day?*

2. We lose muscle mass as we age, which contributes to weight gain and decreased mobility. *Does your weekly workout include resistance exercise, such as weight training?*

3. Weight-bearing exercise is vital for healthy bones, and includes any activity, such as running, walking or tennis, where your body impacts with the ground.
   a) *Do your bones get a workout most days?*
   b) *Are you a healthy weight, i.e. neither under nor overweight?*

4. A healthy diet is crucial for keeping your mind and body young. Fresh fruit and vegetables are bursting with antioxidants and nutrients.
   a) *Do you eat at least five fruit and veg a day?*
   b) *Do you avoid sugar, salt and processed foods?*
   c) *Do you minimize your intake of saturated animal fats and prioritize healthy plant oils?*
   d) *Do you drink plenty of water?*

5. Research shows that stress speeds up cell ageing. *Do you generally avoid stress, and can you cope with stressful situations?*

6. Sun exposure causes premature skin ageing and damages your eyes.
   Do you take precautions to limit the effects of the sun on your body?
   Yes, always – 2 points
   Sometimes – 1 point
   Frankly, no – 0 points

7. Smoking is damaging for your body, including your skin, bones, heart and eyes.
   Are you a non-smoker?
   Yes – 2 points
   I like the occasional cigarette and/or I'm regularly exposed to cigarette smoke – 1 point
   No, I'm a regular smoker – 0 points

8. Excess alcohol damages the liver, heart, your fertility, digestion and bones.
   Do you stick to the government's daily recommended allowance of two to three units a day, or are you teetotal?
   Yes, always – 2 points
   Sometimes – 1 point
   Frankly, no – 0 points

9. Studies show lack of sleep raises inflammatory markers which can contribute to premature ageing.
   Do you get at least six to eight hours of quality sleep a night?

What your results mean...

12 to 16 points – You're holding back the years, as far is humanly possible – keep it up!

8 to 11 points – Overall, your outlook is positive, but try to make a couple of healthy changes.

0 to 7 points – Don't leave the ageing process to fate and your DNA – makes some simple changes to your lifestyle.

THE MEANING OF SUCCESS

Looking youthful doesn't just come from healthy eating and working out. That healthy glow also comes from living the life you want to lead. To do that, you need to define your own version of success.

A great secret to looking and feeling younger is to be happy. This means leading the life you want to lead and not just fulfilling expectations of others. If you are happy with your life, you will be relaxed, less stressed and generally healthier. So how do you get the life you want? A good place to start is to find out what success means to you. Often, without realizing it, we strive for what is considered to be the standard version of success. Family, kids, a good job, lots of money and a large house are all considered the key ingredients of a successful lifestyle. But despite achieving these things, some people find themselves miserable and consequently confused by why they are unhappy. After all, they have 'everything' – so surely they should be happy? Why are they not satisfied? There must be something wrong with them if they aren't happy.

In reality, we all have our own idea of what success should look and feel like, and for many of us it's not necessarily about material things. Of course, most of us like to have nice things, but success isn't solely about having a big house, a flashy car and lots of money. You can have all of those things and be miserable if you're in an unhappy relationship or you hate the job that enabled you to acquire them in the first place.

We don't need to conform to society's definition of what being successful is. Success can't always be measured by money. In fact, if you talk to some of the world's richest people, they will often tell you that money hasn't made them happy. If you're not rich at the moment, you might contradict that statement and say that money would make you happy. But there are downsides to having money. When you are rich, just who can you trust? Are friends your friends because of your money? And how do you keep your money? How do you keep making more of it to maintain your lifestyle? You may have had to work long, unsociable hours to get that money in the first place and had to give up precious time with family and friends. You may have missed family birthdays and other important social occasions in the pursuit of success. And you may also feel the pressure to maintain your success and keep earning more money, so that you are perceived to be continually successful.

HEALTH RISK

Money can also take its toll on your health. Sure, you might be able to afford good healthcare, but the price of getting rich for those who aren't fortunate enough to inherit money is hard work – long hours, in some cases, bad diet, no exercise, and relying on unhealthy vices like smoking and excessive drinking to unwind at the end of another ridiculously long day... ask yourself, is this the kind of life you want for yourself? Is this really what success is about? And, of course, there are examples of very rich people who have died young, who would have traded every penny of their wealth to stay healthy. After all, money may be able to buy the best healthcare, but there are no guarantees when it comes to good health and wellbeing.

THE MEANING OF SUCCESS

In order to get the life you want – the life that will make you feel happy, youthful and vibrant – you need to work out what success means to you. For some, this may mean working part-time and having spare time to spend with their family. For others, it could mean throwing themselves into a job or a career they absolutely love. For some people, it could mean having the time and freedom to travel and explore the world. Others may define success by having less money but more freedom to do the things they want to do.

To get the life you want, you need to first establish exactly what success means to you. Consider the following:

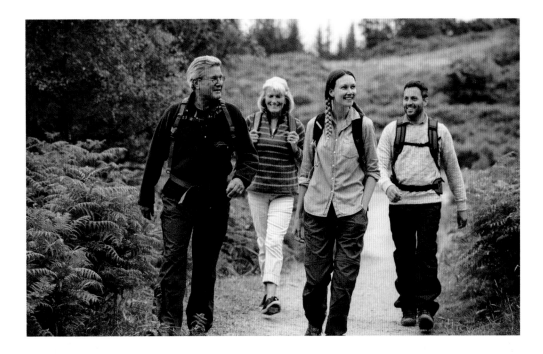

• What are you lacking in your life at the moment? Would you like more time to spend with loved ones, a fresh challenge or new purpose, or the opportunity to do a job that you enjoy?

• What activities do you most enjoy doing? When are you at your most relaxed and content?

• What sort of lifestyle would make you happy? Do you like the idea of a career in an area of business that you love, or would you rather have more downtime? Or would you prefer to have more time to improve your health and fitness?

• Is your current job fulfilling you? If not, what sort of job would you find rewarding?

Write down three things that are most important to you. Also, think about what you haven't done yet. If you were to be told you only had a year to live, what things would be on your bucket list? Once you have answered these questions, start working out how you can have more of these things in your life.

Once you've worked out your own personal definition of success and what makes you happy, you can start thinking about how you can achieve it.

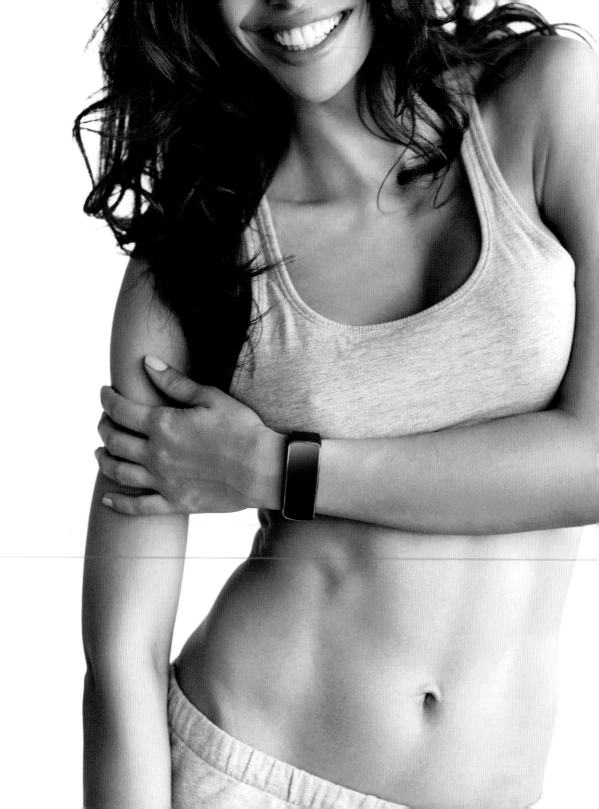

YOUR BODY

Passing years affect every part of our bodies, often in unforeseen ways. This chapter will show your how to maintain health and vitality in every nook and cranny, so you'll feel as young on the inside as you look on the outside. Find out how to look after your teeth, eyes and joints, and take simple steps to protect your fertility, digestion and grey matter.

ALL CHANGE!

Ageing happens so subtly and slowly that you won't even realize it's going on. Here's our guide to how your body alters over the decades...

Believe it or not, your body starts to age from the physical peak of puberty, and we're not just talking about skin; everything from your bone density to muscle mass starts to wane. Happily, there's plenty you can do to slow the speed of change.

IN YOUR 20s

After the hormonal ups and downs of your teens, your skin comes into its own in your 20s. New cells are replicating at an enviable pace, so your complexion should be plump and radiant. Towards the end of the decade, fine lines may start to appear on your forehead and around your eyes, particularly if you haven't been taking care of yourself.

This is likely to be your most carefree decade, but skipping sleep and meals and consuming far too much alcohol can deplete your body.

Your bone density is at its peak in your early 20s, as is your natural aerobic fitness and the amount of lean, metabolism-revving muscle you carry. Even your brain power peaks at age 22. Capitalize on the natural advantages of your age and you'll build sound foundations for the future.
Anti-ageing advice: Now's the time to start a regular and sustained exercise programme to set yourself in good stead and build up credits for the decades to come.

IN YOUR 30s

The natural decline in fitness that started in your 20s may manifest itself now in slight weight gain. The ageing process will also show, albeit faintly on your face. Fine lines will become more evident, your pores may enlarge and your radiance decline. You may notice your first grey hairs.

No part of your body is immune to small changes. You may feel a slight stiffness in your muscles and joints, and they could be more prone to injury. For women, breasts will be less full, and by the time you're 35 your fertility is half what it was at 25. That's not to say you should think of slowing down – quite the contrary!

Anti-aging advice: Your body isn't as resilient as in your 20s, so eat a balanced, healthy diet and keep your weight at a healthy level.

IN YOUR 40s

The fine lines of your 30s may become more pronounced wrinkles, and women may find their skin becoming drier as their bodies enter the perimenopause – the precursor of the menopause, when you still have periods but experience menopause symptoms, such as hot flushes. As levels of the female hormone oestrogen decline, fat will naturally settle on your abdomen and you'll find it harder to shed the pounds.

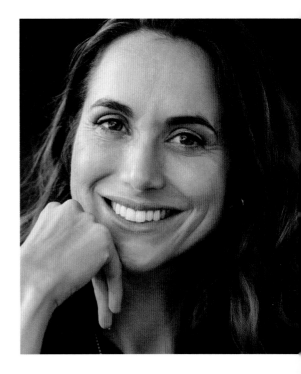

Other changes synonymous with ageing may begin now – for instance, your eyesight and hearing won't be quite as sharp as they once were. Your heart isn't as youthful either. As the decade progresses, it has to work harder to pump blood around your body and your blood vessels lose their elasticity.

Anti-aging advice: Become breast-aware. The incidence of breast cancer increases sharply during your 40s and 50s. Go to www.nhs.uk to find out how to check your breasts.

IN YOUR 50s PLUS

Most women enter the menopause in their early 50s. The menopause can affect your body in many ways. Physically, the drop in oestrogen raises your risk of low bone density, heart disease and breast cancer.

Your skin's hydration levels also dwindle, so it's more prone to sensitivity. And the production of collagen, a protein in the skin responsible for its strength and elasticity, slows down, increasing wrinkles.

If you don't do anything to delay it, other signs of ageing include stiffened joints, hair loss, more fat around the tummy and impaired memory. Your digestive system will be slowing down, making you more prone to constipation, and your senses of taste and smell will decline gradually. Because of wear and tear and a drop in saliva levels, your teeth and gums will also be susceptible.

In your 60s, muscle tissue loss accelerates and, as the cushioning discs between the vertebrae of your spine lose plumpness and depth, your height will also gradually decrease.

Anti-aging advice: Heart disease is your biggest health risk, so eat healthily, exercise regularly and keep cholesterol and blood pressure in check – ask your GP for tests.

THE IMPORTANCE OF HORMONES

Your hormones play a huge part in ageing. Hormones are chemicals that act as messengers between two parts of the body. They influence countless bodily processes, including your metabolism and body clock.

There are various hormone 'factories' in your body – for instance, your pancreas produces insulin – and they slow down as you age.

Your reproductive system relies on complex hormonal activity. The key players in females are: oestrogen, which is involved in the release of eggs from the ovaries; progesterone, which prepares the womb for pregnancy; follicle stimulating hormone; and luteinizing hormone.

At the menopause – usually between the ages of 45 and 55 – levels of oestrogen and progesterone plummet and typical signs of ageing appear. Your skin's elasticity is reduced, your joints may begin to ache and your hair thins. You're also at increased risk of breast cancer, heart disease and osteoporosis. But, as this book explains, you can future-proof your body with a healthy lifestyle.

FIGHTING FIT

Staying young goes further than just changing your skincare routine. Here's how to slow the signs of ageing that you don't see...

We all worry about sagging flesh and body shape changes, but these are only the superficial signs of ageing. Hidden deeper are some serious ageing factors that can affect your long-term health and wellbeing. But just because you can't see them, it doesn't mean you can't do anything to delay these changes. Here's what to do to stay young on the inside!

FERTILITY

Female fertility peaks in your early 20s. According to the Human Fertilisation and Embryology Authority, at 35 you're half as fertile as when you were at 25. Fertility drops dramatically after this – for women aged 35, about 95 per cent who have regular unprotected sex will get pregnant after three years of trying. At 38, only 75 per cent will do so.

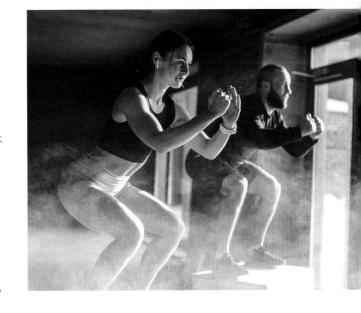

Optimize your fertility with a healthy lifestyle. Being over- or underweight can impair it – in women, a certain level of body fat is needed to regulate the hormones that control ovulation and menstruation, so eat well and exercise. Eat foods rich in folic acid (green leaves), iron (red meat), calcium (dairy), zinc (seafood and asparagus), fibre (brown rice) and unsaturated fat (olive oil). Quit smoking, as this can affect egg formation, ovulation and fertilization,

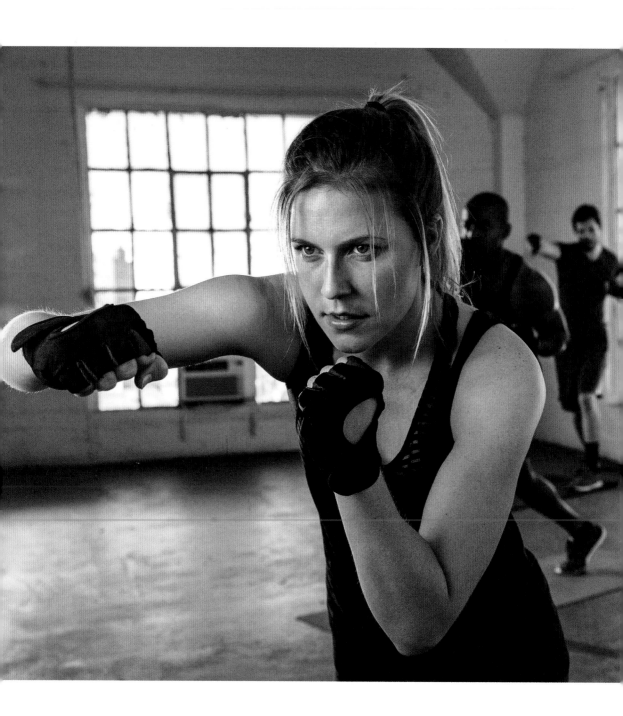

and don't drink alcohol to excess. Stress can impact your reproductive system, so try yoga and meditation.

HEART

A strong heart goes a long way to helping you feel young. It is essentially a muscle, so it will lose strength over time, and as the blood vessels that supply it become less supple, it becomes less efficient. Women's risk of heart disease rises after the menopause because levels of heart-protective oestrogen fall. If you have a family history of heart problems or stroke, be extra aware – the British Heart Foundation recommends you speak to your doctor about your risk from the age of 40 onward. Keep your heart young by following a diet low in salt and saturated fats, and don't smoke or drink excessively, or be a couch potato.

DIGESTION AND KIDNEYS

A well functioning digestive system is key to everything, from healthy skin to good energy levels. Your digestive system slows down over time, but it is possible to keep it young. Drink plenty of water every day and eat lots of soluble fibre. Research shows regular exercise aids digestion and can cut the risk of bowel polyps, which can lead to cancer, by up to 35 per cent. Chew your food well and avoid eating huge meals.

Your urinary system also slows down, as your kidneys reduce in size and weight You're more at risk of urinary incontinence with ageing, but keeping your weight in check and doing pelvic floor exercises can help.

LIVER

Your liver is a chemical processing unit, electricity plant and security guard all rolled into one. The liver performs more than 500 functions, such as breaking down food to make energy, combating infections and neutralizing toxins. It's your largest internal organ and the most resilient – provided you treat it well. Take care of yours by lowering your intake of alcohol and saturated fats. Excess drinking over a long period can cause cirrhosis, while obesity and a bad diet are linked to non-alcoholic fatty liver disease.

VISION ON

Taking care of your eyes can help preserve your sight. Here's how to keep age-related eye problems at bay...

Diminishing eyesight is one of the most frustrating signs of ageing. After the age of 40, our eye muscles weaken and our lenses lose flexibility, so it becomes harder to focus, see smaller objects or read tiny print. However, acute age-related eye problems can be reduced with a healthy lifestyle and regular check-ups. You need an eye test every two years, or more frequently if you wear contact lenses regularly, have diabetes or a family history of eye disease.

> Brightening up your eyes can make you look years younger with little effort.

PARCHED PEEPERS

Your eyes become increasingly dry with age. Air conditioning, contact lenses, cigarette smoke, the menopause and a decline in optical hydration all play a part. This can trigger itching and even blurred vision and light sensitivity. Moisturizing eye drops can help, or ask your optician about 'artificial tear' drops.

Make sure you blink a lot while you're working on a computer and consider buying a humidifier to moisten the air at home. Or try a more drastic treatment – tiny silicone plugs can be temporarily or permanently inserted in the tear ducts to reduce the speed at which your tears drain.

BRIGHTEN YOUR EYES

Your eyes also start to look duller, puffier and bloodshot as you age. Brightening up your eyes can make you look years younger with very little effort or sacrifice. Get plenty of quality sleep, moderate your alcohol intake and avoid cigarette smoke. For an instant lid-lift, apply refrigerated cucumber slices or cold cotton wool pads soaked in rosewater onto your eyes.

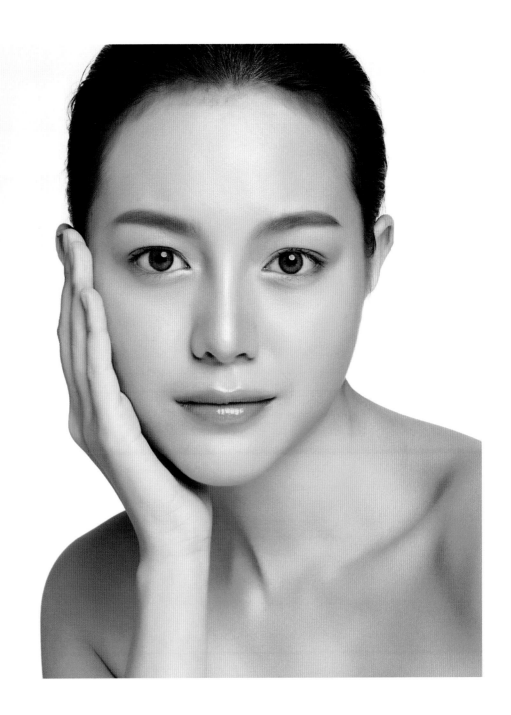

AVOID SUN DAMAGE

Prolonged exposure to sunlight can damage your eyes, especially the retina and lens. Research shows that sun exposure is linked to an increased long-term risk of cataracts – cloudiness in the lens – and

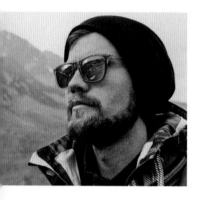

may trigger age-related macular degeneration (AMD), the leading cause of blindness in the UK. Always protect your eyes on sunny days, particularly if you're by the sea or pool, or on a snow-capped mountain – both water and snow reflect glare and can increase the ultraviolet (UV) rays entering your eyes.

Quality sunglasses will also protect the skin around your eyes and prevent eye-scrunching, which can aggravate crow's feet. Look for glasses that offer UVA and UVB protection, with a CE mark or British Standard BSEN 1836:1997, which mean they conform to current recommendations. Protect your eyes with safety goggles during DIY and with sports glasses for activities such as squash.

COSMETIC TRICKS

Make-up can help enhance the youthful appearance of your eyes, or make you look older if you're not careful! Avoid dark, heavily frosted or glittery eye shadow as you age – it can make the whites of your eyes look duller. Think softer, lighter colours with a mild shimmer. As the eyelid skin sags, your eyes can appear smaller. Counteract this by using softer make-up, abstaining from eyeliner on your lower lids and employing a pair of lash curlers to open up your eyes. Get those tweezers out – maintain your natural brow arch to give your eyes a lift.

FEAST YOUR EYES

A startling 65 per cent of us could be at risk of future eyesight problems because we're unaware that what we eat affects our eyes, according to research from the College of Optometrists. Studies show that a balanced diet, rich in antioxidant vitamins A, C and E, lutein (a nutrient) and omega oils may help protect against eye diseases, including AMD. So tuck into leafy greens, (bell) peppers, oranges, blueberries and sweetcorn. Watch your weight too – obesity is linked to eye problems.

JOINT EFFORT

Staying flexible and strong will help you look and feel younger, so start taking care of your bones and joints now!

You may think your bones stop growing in your teens, but they are constantly being renewed, albeit more slowly, in adulthood. Your skeleton actually renews itself every 7 to 10 years.

BOOST YOUR BONES

Bone strength is usually inherited from your parents and in women it declines after the menopause – one in two women over the age of 50 will break a bone, mainly as a result of osteoporosis. However, more controllable factors can contribute – a sedentary lifestyle and excessive exercise, smoking and low levels of vitamin D and calcium all compromise bone density. Even though you build your peak bone mass in your early 30s, it's never too late to strengthen them. A study published in *Medicine & Science in Sports & Exercise* found that, even in postmenopausal women, strength training not only prevented the loss of density, it also built bone matter in the subjects' spine and hips.

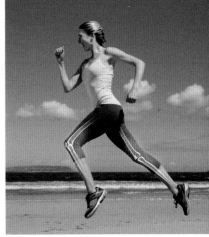

Here are the best ways to boost your bones:

- Stay a healthy weight. Being both under or over your optimum weight can put your bones at risk.
- Exercise regularly. Do weight-bearing exercise, such as jogging, dancing, tennis and power-walking, for at least 30 minutes a day. This will also help you manage stress – high levels of the stress hormone cortisol can damage your bones.
- Eat a calcium-rich diet. Aim for 700 mg a day, equivalent to a 200 ml (½ pint) glass of milk. Leafy greens, tinned fish, fortified cereals and soya foods are other good sources.

- Eliminate your vices. Stick to the daily alcohol limit of two to three units, swap caffeine for herbal teas and drink plenty of water – up to eight glasses a day.
- Get your vitamin D fix. You need this vitamin to absorb calcium, and the best source is sunlight. Aim to get 15 minutes of sun on your skin every day in summer, so your body can store enough for winter.

KEEP YOUR JOINTS YOUNG

We tend to only notice our joints when something goes wrong, but looking after them now will keep you flexible and youthful in the years ahead. Joints become stiff and creaky over time – knees and hips are particular trouble spots because they carry lots of weight.

Age-related inflexibility is down to two major factors – our ability to produce joint-lubricating synovial fluid declines, and cushioning cartilage becomes stiffer and less flexible, so bones may begin to rub together. Minerals may also deposit in and around some joints in a process called calcification.

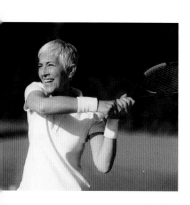

Here's how to keep your joints young and healthy:

- Stay a healthy weight. According to experts, almost 20 per cent of people aged 25 to 34 have a 'joint age' of over 50 because they're carrying excess weight.
- Prioritize exercise. Focus on tennis or yoga, where you shift your body in multiple directions. This will mean your joints will be able to cope better with falls and uneven ground. Weight training also helps strengthen the supportive muscles and ligaments surrounding your joints, so the pressure is taken off them.
- Change your diet. Omega 3 fatty acids in fish oils and pumpkin and sunflower seeds can help reduce the inflammation that may contribute to joint pain. Also, eat leafy greens – a compound found in broccoli and cabbage, called sulforaphane, blocks the enzymes that cause wear and tear on the joints. Although more research is needed to assess its benefits, many people find that glucosamine and chondroitin supplements help ease joint pain.

MIND GAMES

Follow our brain-boosting tips and keep your little grey cells on tip-top form.

Having a lively, active mind is one of the keys to staying youthful. And the good news is that everything from what you eat to who you talk to can help improve your brain function. Age-related brain drain starts so gradually, you may not even notice it happening.

As the number of brain cells (neurons) decreases, even from a fairly early age, nerve impulses sending messages across the brain slow down and our ability to do simple things, such as remembering names and multitasking, wanes. According to research at the University of Virginia in the US, reasoning, spatial visualization and speed of thought decline in our late 20s, and memory begins to dwindle from our late 30s onwards.

But, it's not all doom, gloom and mental confusion. Research shows that keeping fit, healthy and mentally active can slow decline and even stimulate positive changes. In fact, science now shows that we can grow new neurons and neural pathways and regenerate the brain. The cognitive abilities you derive from accumulated knowledge increase up to the ripe old age of 60.

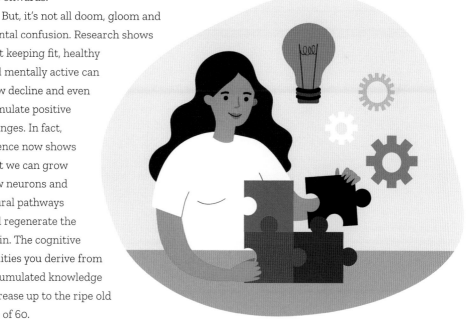

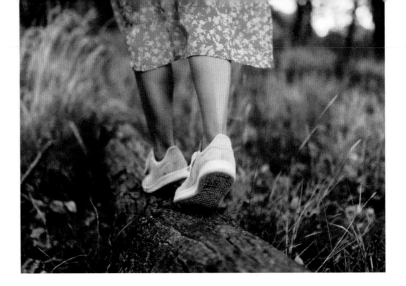

STAY ACTIVE

Regular exercise protects your brain from ageing, as it helps to control blood pressure and weight, both of which influence cognitive functioning as you get older. However, exercise has far more sophisticated benefits too. A Swedish study published in the journal *The Lancet Neurology* found that exercising for half an hour at least twice a week during midlife can reduce the risk of dementia by about 50 per cent. Scientists believe that by boosting circulation, exercise can flush the brain with nourishing blood and oxygen and help keep its complex tissues healthy.

Your exercise programme doesn't have to be adventurous – simple yoga inversions increase blood flow to the brain, and, according to a study led by University of Pittsburgh in the US, simply walking six to nine miles a week can help preserve brain size.

USE IT OR LOSE IT!

Tasks that stimulate your brain can help maintain memory and cognitive processing. A study of cognitively healthy older adults in the *Journal of the American Geriatrics Society* found those who trained their brain were able to improve their auditory information processing speed by about 58 per cent (versus 7 per cent in control subjects).

And you don't need to buy expensive 'brain training' gadgets to keep your mind in eminent condition. A report by *Which?* suggested that crosswords, learning a language, memorizing poetry or playing standard computer games may be as just as effective in stimulating your brain.

STAY SOCIABLE

Proving that good health isn't all about effort and sacrifice, an active social life has been shown to age-proof your brain too. Experts at the Rush University Medical Center in Chicago in the US found that having close friends and staying in contact with family members offers protection against dementia. In fact, the study showed that many people with Alzheimer's who had good social networks didn't suffer from the clinical manifestations of the illness, such as cognitive impairment or dementia. If friends and family don't live nearby, you could join a local group so you feel more part of your community. A running group or regular yoga class will have the added fitness benefits, as well as linking you with like-minded people.

FEED YOUR MIND

While you can't reverse the brain drain with diet alone, experts agree that eating well is phenomenally effective for keeping your grey matter firing on all cylinders. The B vitamins, found in wholegrains and nuts, among other foods, are vital – research at Oxford University recently showed they can halve the rate of brain shrinkage associated with dementia. The much lauded omega 3 oils found in oily fish are also essential – they're high in DHA, a fatty acid thought to support the nervous system. And don't forget that antioxidants such as lycopene (found in tomatoes) and vitamin E (present in nuts, seeds, cereals and eggs) are celebrated for their ability to mop up free radicals. Your brain is a hungry beast, so on a day-to-day basis, don't skip meals or rely on stimulants such as sugar and caffeine. Eat a diet rich in low-GI, slow-energy-release carbs, such as brown rice, to keep it stoked up.

GO GREEN

Drinking green tea could protect your brain against dementia, according to a study by Newcastle University. Green tea contains health-boosting compounds called polyphenols, but scientists didn't know whether they survived the digestion process. The study confirmed that they do survive and also bind to proteins known to play a role in the development of dementia, hence protecting the brain.

PERFECT POSTURE

Want to look instantly slimmer and younger? Just make some simple changes to the way you carry yourself.

One sure way to add years to your appearance is to hunch your shoulders and stand badly. We're naturally more susceptible to twinges in our shoulders, neck and back as we get older. And long-term poor postural habits, such as slouching and hunching, along with a sedentary lifestyle, all combine to make you look older than you really are. But treating your posture with a little TLC won't just ensure you stay enviably mobile and flexible – there is a multitude of additional benefits. Sorting out your posture can help you look slimmer and improve your breathing, so you will look and feel calmer and more confident.

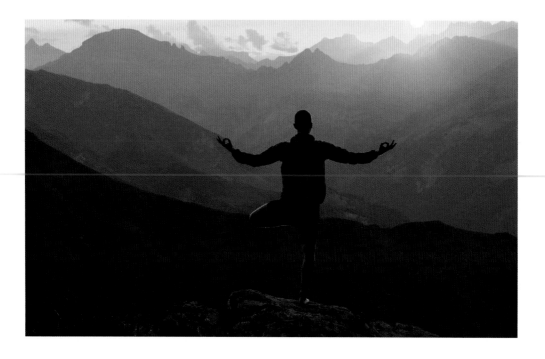

In essence, good posture enables your body to function better. Deskbound jobs, heavy handbags, driving, laptops, phones and sky-high heels – many aspects of modern life – are damaging our posture. Here are some tips on how to behave more courteously towards yours...

WHAT'S YOUR TYPE?

First, discover your posture type by standing sideways next to a mirror to check the position of your pelvis and shoulders. Around 70 per cent of us stand in a sway-back posture with the pelvis tipped back, a result of spending too much time sitting down. Whichever way it's positioned at the moment, you need to bring it back underneath you, in order to keep your spine in alignment.

For those with a sway back, squeeze your bottom and tuck under your tail bone (at the base of your spine), making sure your lower back still retains a gentle curve. Gently pull in your tummy, focusing on the area between your belly button and pubic bone, and check your beltline is horizontal or near to it. Bring your shoulder blades back, then broaden them out down your back as much as you can. Pull your chin in slightly, as though it were being pulled in from the back by a ventriloquist. Your earlobes should be above your collarbone.

STAY SWITCHED ON

Maintain sound posture at all times. From the car to work to the sofa, many of us spend the best part of the day sitting down. It's important to take regular breaks from your recumbent position, but also practise the right

EXERCISES FOR GOOD POSTURE

Head and neck
Create length between your ears and shoulders by lengthening the top of your head towards the sky at all times.

Shoulder girdle
For good shoulder posture, imagine you're sliding your shoulder blades down towards the back of your waist, opening your chest naturally.

Core
Your transversus abdominis muscles are your own built-in corset – to engage them, gently draw your navel to your spine.

Neutral spine
Your lower back should be neither arched nor flattened, but somewhere in between. Maintain your back's natural curves.

Lower body
With your weight in the centre of your feet, draw yourself up, as if creating space between the joints of your ankles, knees, pelvis and spine.

way to align your body when you are sitting to prevent persistent back and neck problems.

Ensure you head is stacked vertically above your sitting bones; jutting it forwards can stress your neck and upper back. Make sure your earlobes stay in alignment with your shoulders. Roll your shoulders back and down. Keep your feet flat on the floor (avoid crossing your legs); your feet should be shoulder-distance apart and knees level with or just below your hips – use a specially designed foot-rest if you need to. Both your hips and knees should be bent at 90 degrees. Try to keep your body soft and don't sit up too stiffly.

WALK TALL

When you walk, hold your head up, bring your shoulders back and pull your tummy muscles slightly in. You're aiming to walk lightly, so shorten and soften your stride. Your head should be tall and not looking down – dropping your head puts a lot of tension on your neck. To see where you're going, drop your eyes without dropping your head.

If you have to carry a bag, make it as light as possible and use alternate sides, or even better, use a backpack so your arms are free. High heels cause your pelvis to tip forward and your head to jut out to compensate for the misalignment. Don't wear them for protracted periods and always choose supportive footwear for walking.

POSTURE FIT

Staying active – in any way – is brilliant for your posture, as it strengthens the muscles that work to support your spine and pelvis. Whichever way you choose to keep fit, maintain a relaxed, open posture and activate your core by imagining you're trying to stop yourself weeing.

For targeted postural benefits, try a holistic mind-body technique. Pilates and yoga are great for working your core, the corset of supportive muscles around your midriff. Meanwhile, Alexander Technique can re-teach you how to sit, stand and walk in an effortless and co-ordinated way. And, according to researchers from Bristol and Southampton universities, it is a bona fide way to manage back pain.

BODY SHAPERS

Try these fashion tips to draw attention from parts of your body you are less comfortable with.

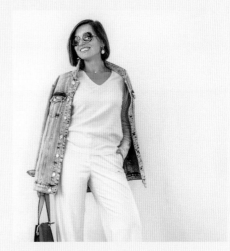

Upper arms
Ditch sleeveless tops along with capped and fitted short sleeves. Three-quarter length and long fluted sleeves are a godsend. Wear a statement bracelet or cuff to emphasize narrow wrists. Men should invest in a uniformly coloured, well-fitted suit in which the jacket's shoulders lie flat.

Chest
If you're well endowed, opt for V-shaped or sweetheart necklines to lengthen your neck. Avoid smock tops and dresses and anything too tight. To draw attention to your bottom half, choose floaty skirts.

Stomach
Shun skinny trousers and pencil skirts. Interesting necklines and chunky necklaces draw the eye upwards. Try low-waisted jeans and flat-fronted trousers or flared skirts to elongate your shape.

Hips and thighs
Go for wide-legged trousers in dark colours. Avoid clingy dresses and boxy, short jackets and tops. Opt for ruffles or bold patterns and jewellery on your top half. Try full-skirted dresses. Wear your jeans in, to improve their fit.

Bottom
Choose wider-legged or flared trousers and jeans, but avoid back pockets. Structured, tailored dresses can sculpt. Draw attention away from your behind with detailing on the front. Wear long-line tops in non-clingy fabrics – go for A-line skirts and coats. Avoid pleats.

Legs
Draw the eye upwards by top-half colour or detail. Avoid shoes with ankle straps. Try maxi-length dresses or shorter hemlines with long boots. For men and women, sharp tailoring on your bottom half is always more flattering than loose styles.

YOUR MIND

It's not just how you treat your body that determines how fast you age – what is going on in your mind plays a big part too. The adage 'you're only as old as you feel' is true, according to experts who found that people who view the ageing process with optimism and confidence are more likely age gracefully. This chapter is about nourishing your mind and soul.

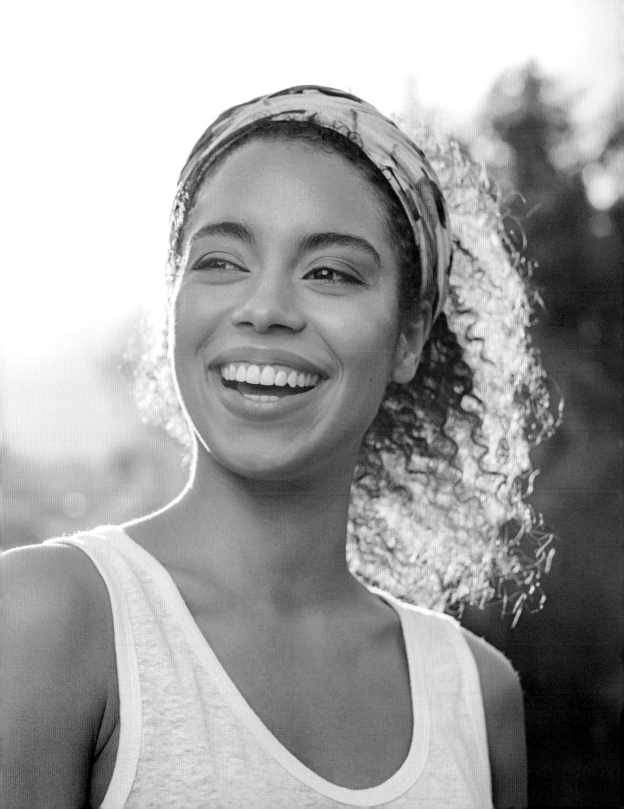

MIND OVER MATTER

Ever feel older than you are? Think again! You can start shedding the years and feeling more vibrant just by changing your attitude to life.

We all know someone whose youthful vitality belies their age. Equally, you're just as likely to have come across people who seem far older than their years. Attitude is everything in the ageing process; it's not just how you treat your body but the way you feel about yourself that than can keep you looking and feeling youthful. Positivity makes you resilient and, according to the latest research, can even have a positive impact on your body at a cellular level. It helps boost your immune system and also helps your body's systems regenerate.

Whether it's because optimism affects us on a biological level or simply encourages sound lifestyle habits, research repeatedly shows buoyant, sociable people are likely to stay healthier for longer. A recent review of more than 160 studies published in *Applied Psychology: Health and Well-Being* on the connection between a positive mental attitude and overall health and longevity has found clear evidence to suggest that happier people enjoy a better sense of wellbeing and longer lives. Here's how to think yourself young...

NURTURE YOUR FRIENDSHIPS

According to research at Brigham Young University in Utah in the US, being lonely can affect your health as adversely as smoking or a bad diet. But by friends, we mean real-life interaction rather through a computer screen; two studies at the University of Arizona have shown cyber relationships don't stave off feelings of loneliness.

LOVE WHAT YOU DO

Studies show that a satisfying work life enriches us, and this includes volunteer work. People who give their time

Research shows buoyant, sociable people are likely to stay healthier for longer.

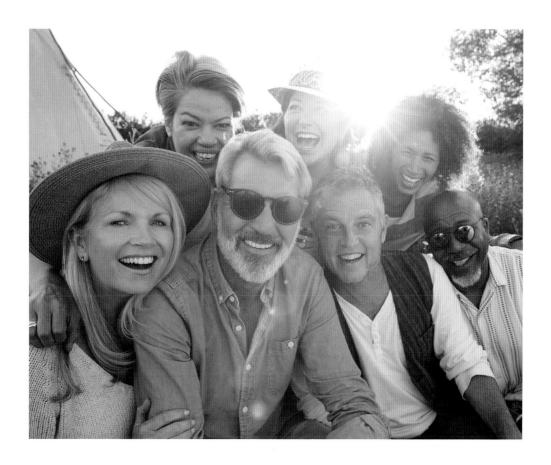

for good causes are proven to have a lower mortality rate and be more physically able to cope with chronic pain or heart disease.

THINK YOURSELF LUCKY

Research by Professor Richard Wiseman at the University of Hertfordshire shows that good luck is a state of mind – and we can maximize our chances of something good happening by creating, noticing and acting on opportunities and listening to our 'gut feelings'. When you're faced with a bad situation, turn it around by imaging how things could have been worse and considering practical solutions.

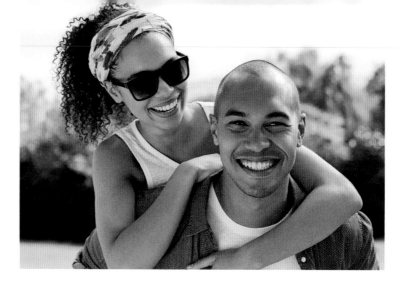

BE FEARLESS

Keep challenging yourself – take risks and get out of your comfort zone every once in a while to push your confidence levels sky-high. It could be as simple as talking to one stranger per day, or as ambitious as changing your career and retraining, travelling to an exotic country or entering a marathon. Whatever it is, just make sure it really tests you. Remember, as we get older, we're more likely to regret the things we haven't done than the things we have.

HAPPY HUGS

Touch is the ultimate anti-ageing sense. Whether it's a hug, massage or holding hands, touch lowers the heart rate, eases pain and even affects our outlook on life. Researchers at Cedars-Sinai Hospital in LA found that Swedish deep massage can trigger measurable changes in the body's immune function. Meanwhile, studies at Yale University show that the feel of objects around us, even those we're sitting on, can affect our behaviour and thought patterns. The softer and more comforting they are, the more likely we are to feel positive. You can also boost your heart health by the simple act of hugging. A team from the University of North Carolina studied the effects of hugging in couples and found it raises levels of oxytocin, the bonding hormone, and reduces blood pressure. So when you feel stressed, reach out – literally!

DE-STRESS, LOOK YOUNGER

Stress doesn't just leave you feeling frazzled. If you're not careful, it can take its toll on your looks and health too.

A little bit of stress never does any harm – in fact, it can spur you into action, making you more productive and zippy. But from your digestion to your hair, your immunity to your heart, in abundance, stress can have tangible effects. On a superficial level, stress triggers bad habits; you're less likely to eat well and may neglect exercise. But it also has biological effects. A University of California study found that sustained periods of stress can add 10 years to the age of a woman's cells. It triggers rushes of a hormone called cortisol, which encourages fat to be laid down around the abdomen, and is detrimental to bone health. Plus, cortisol can accelerate skin ageing; your skin's defence system goes into overdrive, causing inflammation, which can weaken collagen structure, leading to sagginess. According to dermatologists, just two to three months of stress could damage skin and lead to wrinkles. It can also trigger other skin problems, such as acne and eczema.

The odd stressful day probably won't do your looks much harm, but a few angst-filled weeks or months could take their toll. Here's how to take control and de-stress...

UNDERSTAND YOUR MIND

Whether or not you feel stressed comes down to how you perceive a situation rather than what's actually going on. For instance, you might feel terrified at the thought of doing a presentation and lose sleep for weeks beforehand, whereas a colleague will relish the challenge. Being aware of your natural predisposition and what spurs your anxieties is the first step to getting a handle on them. Step back and examine why you find particular situations angst-inducing.

Make a point of de-stressing daily, whether it's a walk in the park or a yoga class.

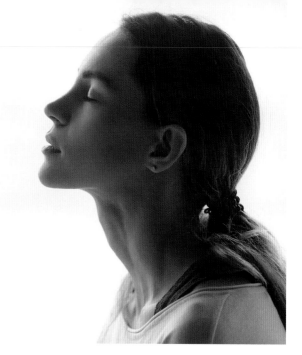

Try to identify your negative thought patterns, such as seeing things in black and white, overgeneralizing or jumping to conclusions. Then consider positive alternatives.

IDENTIFY YOUR PRESSURE PATTERNS

We all have our own repetitive thought patterns — a set way of thinking when we face stressful situations. If you have a need for approval, for example, you'll measure your worth according to what others think of you and feel anxious if you assume you're not up to scratch. If you're a 'catastrophizer', you'll always believe the worst and jump to conclusions, even if you have no evidence to back up your view. Identify and deconstruct your habitual way of approaching issues and ask, is there a healthier alternative?

BECOME STRESS-HARDY

In the midst of a crisis, it can be hard to motivate yourself to do the very things that can help you feel better. Identify your 'back-up' plan — people, activities or commitments that have, in the past, helped you deal better

STRESS WARNING SIGNS

Look out for these symptoms:

- Anger
- Sleep problems
- Lack of motivation and energy
- Headaches
- Muscle tension, aches and pains
- Tightness in the chest
- Skin problems such as eczema
- Poor concentration
- Digestive upset

WHY IS STRESS SO AGEING?

We all know that too much stress is bad for us, but you may not know that it also ages us from the inside. Thousands of years ago, our ancestors faced serious threats to their lives on a regular basis. To them, stress meant being in imminent danger, usually the risk of being eaten by an animal or having to fight others. Nowadays, most of the threats we face are more likely to be emotional or mental stressors. When we face stressful situations, our bodies produce adrenaline in response to a perceived threat and the following processes occur:

- Blood is diverted to the brain, heart, lungs and muscles, which need to work to get you out of danger.
- The heart rate speeds up to pump blood more effectively around the body to these areas.

- Blood is diverted away from the digestive tract, as stopping to eat isn't on the agenda when it's a matter of life or death.
- Breathing speeds up to get oxygen to the muscles as quickly as possible.
- Sweat levels go up to stop the body from overheating.
- Blood sugar levels increase dramatically so that glucose is available to feed the brain and muscles.
- Blood vessels constrict (so blood pressure goes up).
- Your senses become more acute to enable you to pick up as much information as possible in order to make good judgements.
- The body produces the steroid hormone cortisol in response to stress. This makes the stress response last longer, causing long-term health issues.

with stress and feel less isolated. Do you have a friend whose energy is infectious? Or do you have a favourite walk that lifts your spirits? Think ahead about the tools you can use in an emergency.

SMALL CHANGES

To prevent long-term accumulation of anxiety, make a point of de-stressing daily, whether it's a walk in the park, deep breathing or an evening yoga class. Always take a break from your desk, even if it's only for 10 minutes, and avoid skipping meals. Watch your posture and body language – smile and laugh as much as you can; research shows this can have a positive effect on your health.

BREATHE YOURSELF BETTER

Balance your active life with plenty of chill-out time.
Breathing well paves the way to a younger body.

We breathe so instinctively – more than 23,000 times a day, in fact – that
most of us have forgotten how to do it properly and take our lungs for
granted. But using the full might of your lungs can bestow age-defying
benefits, including increased levels of confidence, energy and calm – and,
studies show, lower blood pressure. This all helps to keep the wrinkles
at bay. We're hard-wired from birth to breathe deeply and use our full
lung capacity, engaging the diaphragm and intercostal muscles (between

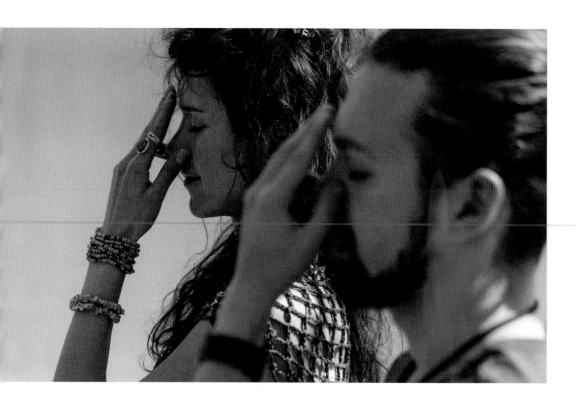

the ribs), but, over time, our breath tends to become shallower. Breathing poorly results in low energy levels and poorly nourished cells. Stress is partly to blame – and it's a vicious circle because restricted breathing increases anxiety further. Here's how to breathe yourself better and younger...

MINDFUL BREATHING

Re-teach yourself how to breathe from your belly, not your chest, pushing out your lower abdomen gently while inhaling and returning it on the exhale. Also, concentrate on breathing through your nose rather than your mouth, as your nose acts as an air filter.

BOOST YOUR LUNG POWER

Your lung capacity declines dramatically by the time you reach your 70s, as your respiratory muscles lose strength, your rib cage becomes less flexible and the alveoli, the tiny grape-like sacs of your lungs, start to thin and become less efficient at processing oxygen and carbon dioxide. You can protect your lungs and maximize your breathing from a young age by not smoking, taking plenty of aerobic exercise and wearing a mask if you're doing DIY or exposed to fumes and vapours.

- Breathe in and out of your feet, figuratively speaking. On an out breath, visualize roots growing down from your feet and into the floor – this helps ground you and slow down racing thoughts. Remove obvious physical tension in your body by shrugging your shoulders and uncrossing your arms and legs.
- Breathe in stages. Imagine your abdomen is made up of different parts and inhale from your lower abdomen to your chest for a count of four. Then exhale from your nose to the count of nine. Breathing out for longer than you breathe in helps trigger your body's instinctive relaxation mechanism.
- Spot-check your breathing patterns throughout the day, but also devote some time to looking after your lungs, particularly if you're prone to stress. T'ai chi and yoga focus on breathing and have added fitness benefits. Try meditation too; research published in the *Journal of Neuroscience* shows that those who practised meditation for a five-year period had a biological age of around 12 years younger than their real age.

GET YOUR BEAUTY SLEEP!

We've all heard the benefits of having enough sleep. Here's how to ensure you get a good night's rest...

It's not called 'beauty sleep' for nothing! Sleep is essential for beautiful, glowing skin and helping your body stay at its peak. When you sleep, your body produces growth hormones, vital for cell renewal. We've all noticed the dull skin and hollow eyes we get after a bad night's sleep. A study at Karolinska Institute in Stockholm found chronically sleep-deprived people appeared less attractive and unhealthier than those who were well rested. Lack of sleep not only weakens the immune system, it's implicated in a variety of conditions, including heart disease, stroke, diabetes and depression – none of which will help you feel youthful! To stay looking and feeling energized and young, you need to aim for a regular, set amount of good-quality shut-eye. Here's how to do it...

HOW MUCH IS ENOUGH?

Don't get hung up on how much sleep you need – it's all about quality, not quantity. Everyone's different (average sleep time varies from six to eight hours or more), so listen to your body and work out the optimum amount of time you feel you should sleep for.

GET INTO A ROUTINE

Maintain regular sleeping times, even at weekends, to send strong messages to your body clock and wean it off alarms. When you wake up in the morning, make sure you get a 10-minute dose of direct daylight to help set your body clock.

HAVE A NAP

If you're a good sleeper and it's practical to do so, take a recharging catnap during the natural afternoon slump. But don't snooze for longer than 20 minutes or you'll enter deep sleep and feel worse afterwards.

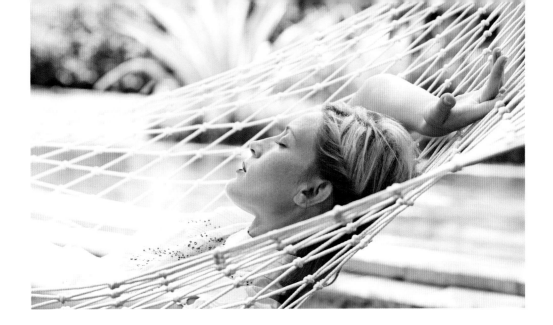

CREATE A RESTFUL SPACE

Ensure your boudoir is conducive to sleep. Get a good-quality mattress and bedding, keep your laptop, phone and TV out of the room, declutter, darken and cool the space – the optimal temperature is from 16°C to 18°C.

WIND DOWN BEFORE BED

Avoid pre-slumber stimulants, such as scary films, high-impact exercise, caffeine, alcohol and heavy meals (sex is fine, as it's also relaxing). Try some wind-down tools to help beat insomnia, including meditation, a warm bath, a warm, milky drink or camomile tea and an undemanding paperback. Spritz your pillow with a calming aromatherapy blend that includes lavender, and empty your mind of stressful thoughts – have a notebook beside your bed and note down a to-do list for the next day if necessary.

LIGHTS OUT

If you find it hard to nod off, invest in some blackout curtains to block out street lights. Keep your home lighting soft before you wind down for bed and always switch off any light sources before you hit the pillow.

Sleep is about quality, not quantity, and everyone is different, so listen to your body.

YOUTH-BOOSTING YOGA

We've picked the best age-defying and gravity-defying yoga poses to help you look young and stay super-flexible.

We're all familiar with the stress-busting, body-shaping benefits of yoga, but studies show it can also protect your body from age-associated illnesses. Following a regular yoga practice can help reduce the body's inflammation response, implicated in arthritis, heart disease and stroke, among other illnesses. You can find some of the most popular anti-ageing poses on the following pages.

Studies show regular yoga practice can protect your body from age-associated illnesses.

FIND YOUR STYLE

Confused by the multitude of yoga styles out there? Although there are bedrock postures, the speed and intensity of classes varies greatly. If you're a novice, even if you consider yourself to be very fit, start with a gentle form, such as hatha or Iyengar. Here are the common types:

IYENGAR Slow and precise, this style encourages you to use accessories such as belts to aid postures.

HATHA An umbrella form, so classes tend to include a mix of asanas, breathing exercises and meditation, and go at a manageable pace.

ASHTANGA Gymnastic and speedy, so it has an aerobic element. Classes are comprised of a precise set of asanas that flow together, so you're rarely still.

BIKRAM 26 traditional asanas, performed quickly and in a very hot room. Definitely not for novice yogis!

KUNDALINI An expressive form focusing on meditation, chanting and breathing.

BEFORE YOU BEGIN...

Wait four to five hours after a heavy meal, around two hours after a snack. Practise in loose-fitting clothes and bare feet.

- Always work on a non-slip mat. Use blocks, bolsters and belts to assist your practice, where appropriate.
- Although you should feel challenged during the poses, you shouldn't be in any pain. Ease yourself into each pose.
- Breathe slowly and calmly, inhaling and exhaling through your nose.
- Avoid inverted poses if you're menstruating, have or are recovering from head and neck injuries, have glaucoma or high blood pressure.

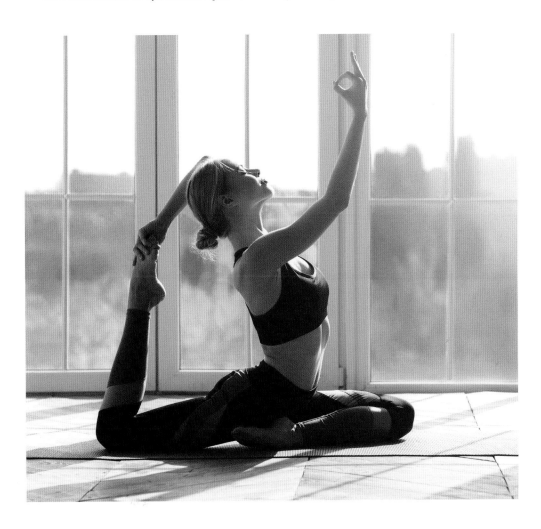

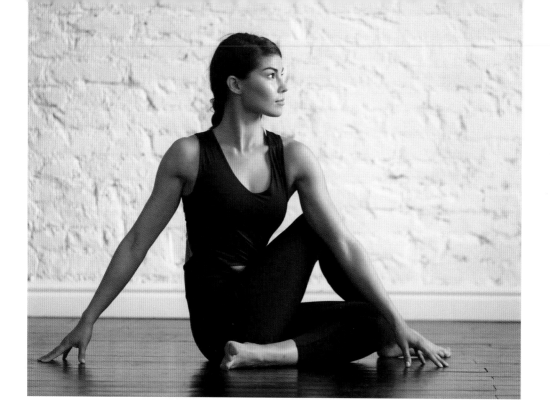

Seated twist

This stretches and restores your body and kick-starts your digestion.

- Sit cross-legged with your arms at your sides, fingertips touching the floor.
- Inhale, elongating your spine upwards. Then, as you exhale, twist gently to the right, place your left hand on your outer right thigh and place your right hand on the floor behind you with your fingertips facing back.
- Look over your right shoulder and hold for 20 to 30 seconds. With each exhalation, gently twist a little more. Repeat on the other side.

Sphinx

Brilliant for stretching your spine and chest.

- Lie face-down on a mat, with your legs together. Tuck your elbows in, and lay your forearms on the ground, hands pointing forward.

- Keeping your hands directly underneath your shoulders, inhale and press down with your palms and forearms, then lift your chest and head so you're looking straight ahead. Broaden out your chest and lift your ears away from your shoulders.
- Hold for 20 to 30 seconds, then exhale and return to the start. Repeat.

Tree

Builds strength in your legs, feet, bottom and core muscles.
- Stand with your feet together. Moving your bodyweight onto your right foot, catch your left ankle and place the sole of your left foot on the inside of your right thigh. If that's too challenging, place it on your calf, but avoid your knee joint altogether.
- Place your hands in prayer position in front of your chest and look straight ahead.
- Hold, then inhale and extend your arms overhead, palms facing each other. Join your palms, without bending the elbows. Hold for 20 to 30 seconds, then repeat on the other leg.

Downward dog

Energizes you, boosts your complexion and strengthens your upper body.
- From all fours (hands and knees on the mat), curl your toes under and push back, raising your hips and straightening your legs. Your feet should be hip-distance apart, fingers spread and hands shoulder-width apart.
- Move your shoulder blades away from your ears. Let your head hang. Engage your legs strongly. Keep your tail bone high, so you're in an inverted 'V' shape and sink your heels towards the floor. Stay for 20 to 30 seconds, then bend your knees and come down.

The Downward Dog pose stretches your body while strengthening your core and improving circulation.

Camel

Stretches your upper body and builds flexibility in your spine. Boosts your digestive and reproductive systems.

- Kneel on the floor with your knees and feet parallel and hip-width apart, pressing your shins and the tops of your feet onto the floor. Rest your hands on your hips and gently arch your back, moving your tail bone forward, but keeping your thighs perpendicular. Move slowly.
- When you're ready, reach down and place your right palm on your right foot. If this is enough for you, stay here, then come up and repeat on the left. Or, if you feel comfortable, place both hands down at the same time.
- Keep your neck in a neutral position or drop your head back. Stretch open your chest. If you can't touch your feet without compressing your lower back, turn your toes under to lift your heels. Stay here for 30 seconds to a minute.
- To release, place your hands on your hips, inhale and lift your head and chest, leading with your heart.

The Camel pose is a great antidote to sitting or leaning forward – it bends the spine in the opposite direction and improves your posture.

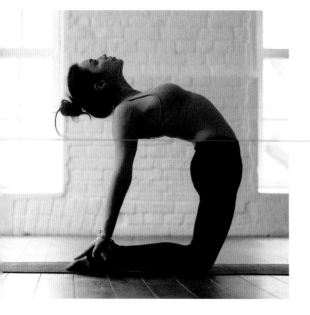

Inverted L

Boosts circulation and relieves tired legs.

- Sit sideways to a wall, placing your hips as close to the skirting board as possible.
- Swivel your body around, so your legs are resting up against the wall, with your feet hip-distance apart.
- Take your arms over your head (palms upwards), and relax. If this arm position is uncomfortable, rest your arms out to the sides, palms up.
- Close your eyes and breathe deeply for 30 seconds to one minute.
- To release, bend your legs, return your arms to your sides and tip onto your side. Don't stand up too quickly or you could get a head rush.

Warrior and side angle

Opens your hips and strengthens your legs, bottom and arms. Boosts knee flexibility.

- From a standing position, step or jump your feet around 1.2 m (4 ft) apart, raising your arms to shoulder height.
- Turn your right foot slightly in and your left foot 90 degrees out. Keep your torso – including your hips – facing straight ahead.
- Exhale, and bend your left knee to a right angle, keeping your right leg straight. Hold for 20 to 30 seconds; this is Warrior II.
- From here, exhale and place your left forearm on your left thigh and raise your right arm overhead, palm facing the floor.
- Look up to the ceiling and hold for 20 to 30 seconds. Inhale and rise back to Warrior II.
- Exhale and straighten your left leg. Repeat on the right side.

Lion

Releases tension and stretches the muscles in your face and neck.

- From a kneeling position, place your palms on the floor in front of your knees, with fingers spread.
- Elongating your chest and tucking your tail bone in, look up to the ceiling and open your mouth. Stick out your tongue and roar as you exhale.
- Release the pose after one full breath, and repeat two or three times.

Child

Eases out your neck and back, and calms your mind.

- Sit on your heels with your knees apart and big toes touching.
- Inhale, then, as you exhale, bring your forehead to the floor and let your arms rest by your sides, palms facing the ceiling.
- Relax here for as long as you like, breathing gently.

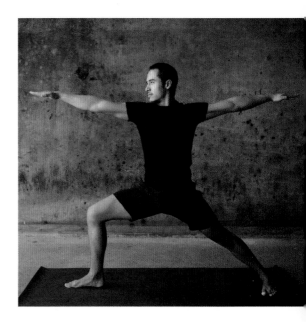

The Warrior II pose creates a good stretch in your hips and enhances your strength, flexibility and stamina.

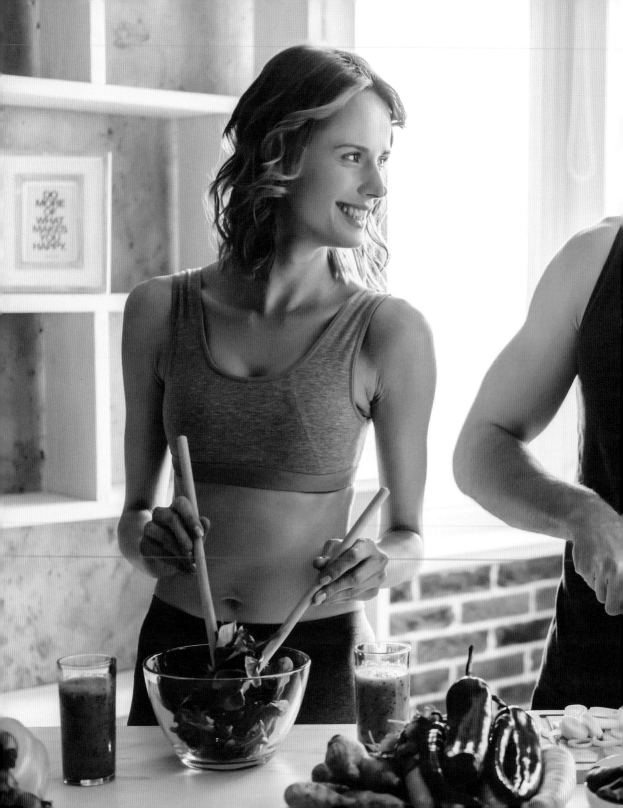

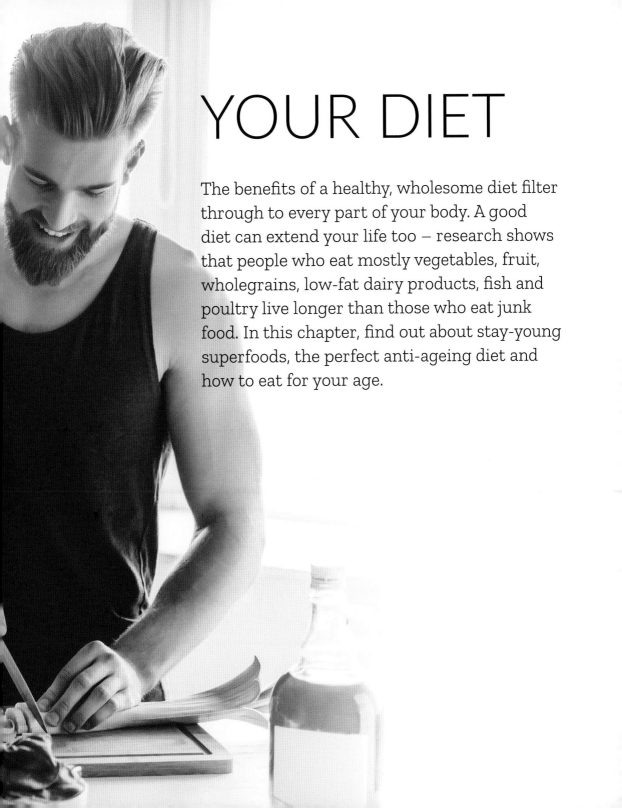

YOUR DIET

The benefits of a healthy, wholesome diet filter through to every part of your body. A good diet can extend your life too – research shows that people who eat mostly vegetables, fruit, wholegrains, low-fat dairy products, fish and poultry live longer than those who eat junk food. In this chapter, find out about stay-young superfoods, the perfect anti-ageing diet and how to eat for your age.

YOUTH STARTS ON THE INSIDE

If you want to look younger, you can't ignore the quality of the foods you put into your body. Here's why a good diet is crucial to looking younger...

EASY WAYS TO IMPROVE YOUR DIET

- Don't have any junk in the fridge. If you buy cakes or chocolate for a 'friend', buy them on the way to visit the friend. Having treats in the house will only lead to temptation, especially if you've had a stressful day, as you'll convince yourself that you 'deserve' a treat.
- Plan ahead. Make sure the fridge is stocked with healthy foods like fruit and veg. If you end up throwing veg away, consider buying frozen veg instead.
- Prepare your own food. That way, you'll know exactly what's in the food you eat.
- Don't eat out more than once a week. There are lots of extra calories in restaurant food and portion sizes tend to be bigger too, which means you could easily gain weight. Make it an occasional treat only.
- If you drink alcohol, be sure to drink plenty of water as well. This will help you stay hydrated and prevent your skin from drying out.

You are what you eat. It's a simple fact. While the occasional treat in moderation should be fine if we eat healthy foods most of the time, eating a constantly bad diet can lead to your skin and teeth ageing prematurely. We all know that sugar can cause dental decay, encouraging bacteria and discoloration of teeth, but it can also damage the skin's collagen. Too much alcohol can age us in various ways. Apart from affecting our quality of sleep, which in itself can prevent the body from repairing well, it can also cause dehydration, leading to dry skin. In addition, it can lead to toxins building up in the liver, which can give you bad skin, including acne and wrinkles.

A good skincare routine will help you look younger, but when it comes to protecting your skin, you need to eat the right foods. What you put into your body will have a direct effect on your facial appearance. For instance, according to some GPs, middle-aged women who have young-looking skin eat a lot of vitamin C. Vitamin C builds collagen, which is the structure that keeps your skin looking smooth.

GOOD SKIN GUIDE

The skin is the body's largest organ, and a good diet will help the appearance of your skin. Vitamins A, C and D will help to protect your skin from ultraviolet light. Vitamin A is also essential for good vision, as well as a healthy immune system, and a diet high in vitamin A will help with heart health. Vitamin A is also taken in supplement form for acne and various skin conditions, including wrinkles. Foods containing vitamin A include carrots, apricots, nectarines, spinach and broccoli.

Vitamin C is needed to repair tissues in the body, including the skin. Good sources of vitamin C include oranges, grapefruit, cauliflower, broccoli, strawberries and pineapple.

Vitamin D, found in fish like herring, mackerel, sardines and tuna, could help to prevent or reduce the risk of high blood pressure and high cholesterol. It's also good for skin and can boost the immune system.

The more you delve into the topic of nutrition and anti-ageing, the more you realize that you can't escape the fact that a healthy diet is one of the best ways to look younger. Other foods that help prevent ageing skin include:

Kale – This dark green leafy superfood contains vitamin K, which helps to improve circulation, giving your skin a healthy glow.

Eggs – Experts believe that the lean protein contained in eggs can provide building blocks for collagen.

> A study found that people who ate diets high in vitamin C were less prone to wrinkles.

Tomatoes – These contain lycopene, an antioxidant that helps fight free radicals (molecules that damage your cells, including skin cells), which can lead to premature ageing.

Red (bell) peppers – These are rich in vitamin C, which can help to reduce the appearance of wrinkles. A study published in the *American Journal of Clinical Nutrition* found that those people who ate diets high in vitamin C were less prone to wrinkles.

Fats and oils – Adding the right oils and fats to your diet, along with eating healthy foods like nuts and some fish, will help your oil-producing glands work efficiently, which will help to prevent skin from drying out. Sadly, our skin gets drier as we age due to a decrease in sebum (this produces moisture naturally). Other ways to get more oils in your diet include using extra virgin olive oil and coconut oil (the latter in moderation). Oily fish like trout, salmon and mackerel are also good choices for keeping your skin moisturized.

Green tea – This cleansing tea contains astaxanthin, a carotenoid that improves the elasticity of the skin and therefore helps achieve a younger appearance.

YOU ARE WHAT YOU EAT

It's no surprise that what you put in your body has a big impact on its outward appearance. Here's our pick of the top ten anti-ageing foods...

Wrinkly skin and old age usually go hand in hand. In fact, wrinkles are often viewed as an unavoidable part of the ageing process. But the truth is, there are ways in which we can slow this process – and in some cases even reverse part of the damage – simply by taking into consideration the body's nutritional needs. One factor that can considerably speed up the ageing process is an excessive production of free radicals and the onset of oxidative stress. Unbeknown to many, a high concentration of oxygen is actually toxic and can have a corrosive effect on our cells. Dangerous by-products – free radicals – are produced during bodily processes that use oxygen, such as the combination of oxygen with digested food. If these pesky molecules are in abundance (oxidative stress), then the ageing process is accelerated and the onset of age-related diseases, such as arthritis, cancer, Parkinson's, premature ageing and stroke, to name just a few, is more likely. You can see a similar process happening if you cut an apple in half and leave it uncovered – the browning that occurs is oxidization. Without protection, the apple will soon rot away.

Free radicals will always be produced naturally within the body, and, in fact, some oxidation action is necessary for life. However, environmental factors, such as industrial chemicals found in plastics and foods, cigarette smoke, excessive exposure to the sun (UV rays), pollution, excessive exercise, pesticides used in farming and an unhealthy diet (one that's lacking in antioxidants and is high in processed foods) all contribute to the production of these damaging molecules.

In order to keep free radicals under control, the body is able to produce antioxidants. Antioxidants stop the 'rusting' of your cells by reacting with the free radicals before they have a chance to do any

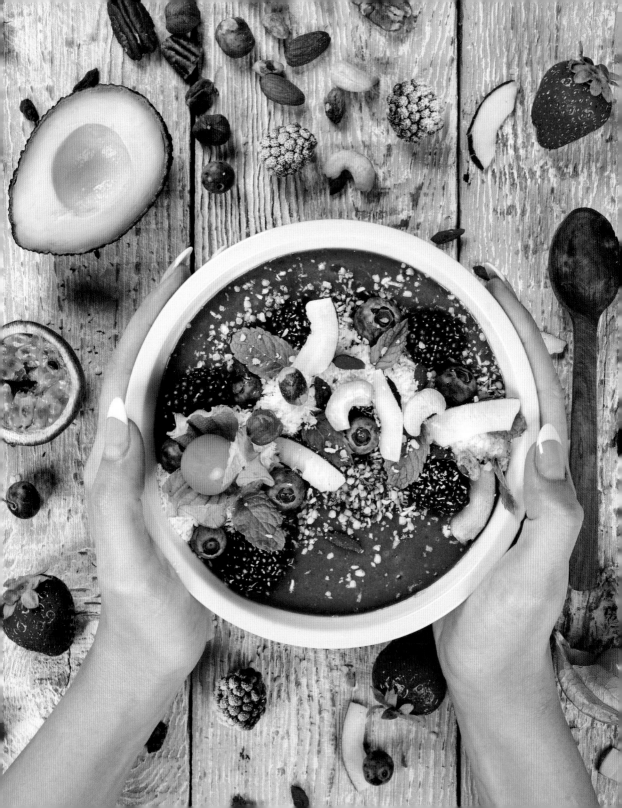

damage. The problem is that, in cases of oxidative stress, where there are too many free radicals being created, the body cannot produce enough antioxidants on its own. This is why we simply must include antioxidant-rich foods within our diet if we want to age well from the inside out. We now know antioxidants (along with their phytonutrient and carotenoid groups) are major players when it comes to protecting our youthful looks, but if we really want to maintain a life-long glow, a whole host of nutrients can help out. So what exactly should you be eating to protect and enhance youth? Here are our ten top anti-ageing picks...

1. SALMON

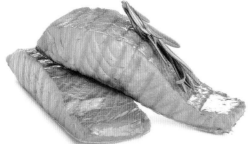

This oily fish houses a type of phytonutrient called astaxanthin, which may help to protect the skin against UV damage and prevent premature ageing. It's also been found to contain small bioactive protein molecules that are said to support joint cartilage.

Salmon is a great source of protein, which is important for bone health.

2. SWEET POTATOES

Vitamin A can prevent dry and flaky skin by stopping a build-up of old keratin cells. Sweet potatoes are the highest vitamin A-containing plant food available. Eating them regularly should also help to support your immune system and vision.

3. LEAFY GREEN VEGETABLES

Dark, leafy greens, such as kale and Swiss chard, are rich in vitamin K, which is partly responsible for bone density. You'll also find various forms of vitamin A in your dark green veg – vital for maintaining eye health.

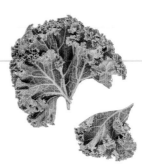

4. PINK GRAPEFRUIT

This is rich in vitamin C, which helps to produce collagen and prevent free-radical damage from cigarette smoke and UV rays. Vitamin C may also soothe symptoms of conditions such as rheumatoid arthritis.

Sugar is demonized for contributing to a host of serious health conditions, but it can also have a major effect on skin health. Too much sugar can cause sugar molecules and protein molecules to 'cross-link', producing harmful new products. This process is called glycation. These harmful new molecules may result in wrinkling, along with loss of elasticity, stiffness and accelerated ageing.

As well as avoiding sugars, salt and processed white foods, try to moderate salt and your intake of red meat – studies have linked an excess consumption of red meat to heart disease and cancers, including bowel and breast cancer.

Also watch your intake of saturated animal-derived fats, such as butter, and hydrogenated or trans-fats, which are artificially created fats present in fast food, some margarines and mass-produced baked goods.

Choose healthy methods of cooking, such as grilling and steaming, and eat charred, barbecued foods in moderation, as these contain carcinogenic compounds.

5. POPCORN

This tasty snack is incredibly high in polyphenols – micronutrients that have been strongly linked to preventing heart disease and some cancers. Avoid versions coated in butter, sugar or salt – instead, pop your own and dust with cinnamon.

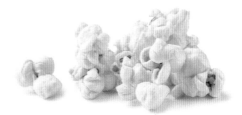

6. FLAXSEED OIL

This oil shouldn't be heated, as this can destroy its delicate essential fats, but it should be drizzled over salads or cooked vegetables. It contains alpha lipoic acid – an antioxidant that can actually regenerate and recycle other antioxidants!

As well as being high in antioxidants, popcorn is a good source of fibre.

7. COCONUT OIL

The benefits of coconut oil are plenty: hair and skincare, stress relief, cholesterol-level maintenance, weight loss, improved immune system, better digestion and regulated metabolism. It's also antimicrobial, antioxidant, antifungal and antibacterial. What's not to love?

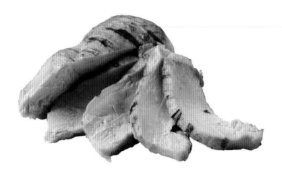

8. TURKEY

Turkey is not only a great source of collagen-boosting protein, but it also contains tryptophan, an amino acid that has been said to aid sleep – vital for glowing skin and a youthful appearance.

Turkey is highly nutritious, supplying all the amino acids that we need for growth and repair.

9. EGGS

Egg yolks are high in a nutrient called choline, which is required for a complicated process within our bodies called methylation. Deficits in methylation have been linked to memory loss and cardiovascular disease, so eat up!

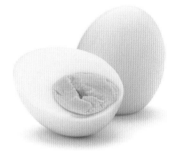

10. PUMPKIN SEEDS

Try sprinkling a tablespoon of pumpkin seeds over porridge, yogurt or salads to boost your daily intake of zinc. Often overlooked, this essential mineral is needed for new skin cell production as well as preventing stretch marks.

SUPPLEMENT YOUR ANTI-AGEING DIET

You can boost your diet by trying some of the following anti-ageing herbs:

Amla (Indian gooseberry) is an ayurvedic herb, rich in vitamin C and antioxidants. As a tincture, take 30 drops up to three times a day.

Milk thistle can help support healthy liver function and the elimination of toxins – try it in either tablet or tincture form.

Gingko biloba has long been used to treat circulatory disorders and boost memory.

Ginseng is revered for its rejuvenating and stimulating effects, and research shows it can help prevent free-radical damage, but avoid it if you suffer from high blood pressure.

Dong quai root (angelica) helps maintain healthy hormone balance and is a popular supplement during the menopause.

EAT FOR YOUR AGE

Here is a handy decade-by-decade healthy eating guide for a slim and youthful body.

An age-appropriate diet can help you stay feeling and looking your best while laying down good health foundations to meet the challenges of the next decade. Here's how to eat your way to a healthy head start in the anti-ageing stakes...

IN YOUR 20s

This is the time to capitalize on your body's natural good health. Your bone density, muscle mass and metabolism peak in your 20s, so treat them with respect and build up a bank of reserves for the future. To feed your bones, eat a wide range of calcium-rich foods, including dairy and tinned fish. To bolster your muscles, pack in healthy protein, such as eggs, nuts, pulses, tofu and lean meat. Iron deficiency is common in young women – leafy greens, dried fruit and red meat should redress the imbalance, or see your GP for advice. This is likely to be your party-hard decade, so watch your alcohol intake – it's calorie-laden, dehydrating and can disturb your sleep. Try not to skip meals or overdo takeaways – fast food needn't be unhealthy if you sharpen your cooking skills. Balanced, regular meals will keep your mood and energy levels constant.

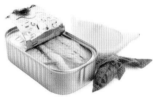

IN YOUR 30s

Prevent the natural decline of muscle mass (and slowing metabolism) by eating plenty of protein. Women can maximize their fertility by keeping alcohol to a minimum and eating folate-rich foods, including leafy greens and fortified wholegrains. Start looking after your heart. Swap saturated fats for plant oils, reduce your salt intake and increase your fibre consumption. Watch your weight as it'll get harder to shed the pounds as you age. Stock up on

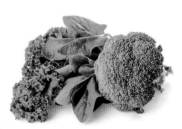

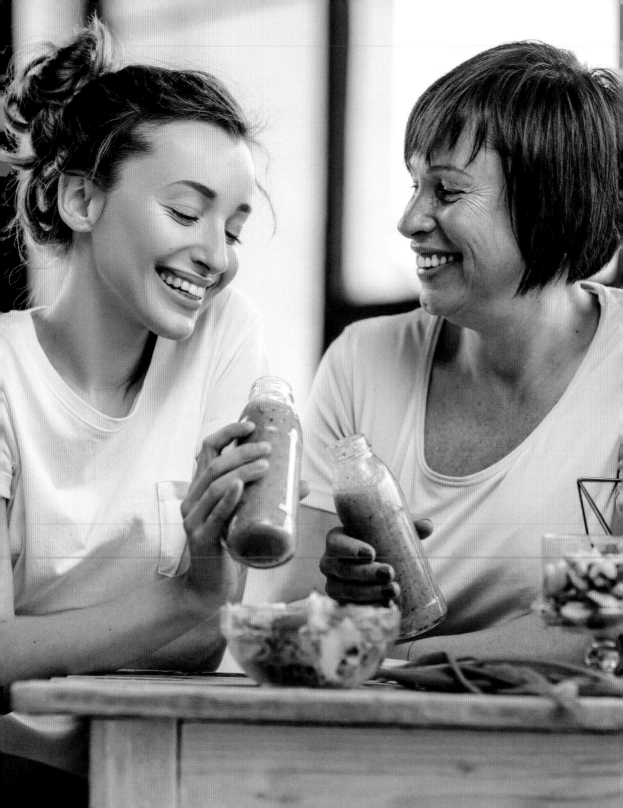

healthy essentials such as brown rice, pasta, tinned tomatoes and pulses, nuts and seeds. Fine lines can show in this decade, so make sure your diet is brimming with antioxidants — available in green tea and brightly coloured fruit and veg.

IN YOUR 40s

The pounds can creep on in your 40s, especially around your belly. This happens as muscle mass dips; levels of oestrogen go down in women, and testosterone production is reduced in men, both of which encourage weight to gather in your midriff. As well as resistance training, a balanced diet will help counteract this. Watch your portion sizes — you need fewer calories with each decade as your metabolic rate slows. Maximize your metabolism with regular meals, and eat lean protein and low-GI carbohydrates, such as wholegrains. Along with fruit and veg, wholegrains will ensure you get enough fibre to protect your heart and your digestive system. Women's risk of breast cancer increases, so minimize alcohol and, as the menopause approaches, get enough calcium and vitamin D to nourish your bones. Include phytoestrogens in your diet — available in soya products — as they can help recoup some of your body's natural decline in oestrogen.

IN YOUR 50s PLUS

Following a healthy diet from a young age pays dividends now — but it's never too late to change. What you eat now can delay age-related diseases, such as dementia, and could reduce your risk of certain cancers, including bowel and breast. After 55, you have a greater risk of atherosclerosis, where the blood vessels lose elasticity and start to clog, increasing your risk of stroke and heart attack. Continue to eat a cardio-friendly diet. Packing your diet with fruit and veg, fibre-rich foods and lean proteins will also help you maintain a healthy weight, which will lighten the load on your joints and reduce your risk of type 2 diabetes. Probiotic yogurts or drinks will help replenish levels of gut bacteria.

LOOK YOUNGER IN 7 DAYS

Try our healthy meal plan to boost your energy levels, improve your skin and make your eyes sparkle.

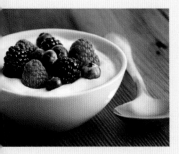

Day 1:
BREAKFAST
Berries, yogurt and pumpkins seeds

Combine fresh blueberries and raspberries with 120 g (4 oz) low-fat live natural yogurt and some pumpkin seeds.
Benefits: Berries are high in vitamin C, which help protect your skin from free-radical damage. Pumpkin seeds are high in omega 6 oils to keep your skin moisturized.

SNACK
Fresh gazpacho and almonds

Blend half a cucumber, four tomatoes, half a red (bell) pepper, one garlic clove, two spring onions (scallions) and fresh basil with one tablespoon each of olive oil and red wine vinegar. Sieve and add water to get the consistency you like. Serve cold, topped with flaked almonds.
Benefits: Raw veg are packed with antioxidant vitamins and minerals. Almonds are a source of essential fats that help build skin cells and heal blemishes.

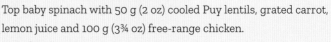

LUNCH
Grilled chicken and Puy lentil salad

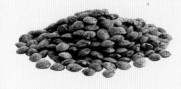

Top baby spinach with 50 g (2 oz) cooled Puy lentils, grated carrot, lemon juice and 100 g (3¾ oz) free-range chicken.
Benefits: Lentils and chicken are a good source of selenium – great for healthy skin and hair.

SNACK
Balsamic strawberries with mascarpone cheese

Marinate 100 g (3¾ oz) strawberries with 1 tsp balsamic vinegar, and mix in mascarpone with low-fat live natural yogurt.

Benefits: The yogurt provides your gut with friendly bacteria to aid digestion and boost your skin.

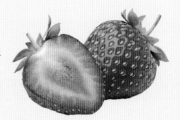

DINNER
Roast salmon with roasted tomatoes

Pre-heat your oven to 180°C/gas mark 4. Place the salmon and tomatoes on a baking tray and roast on the middle shelf for 10–12 minutes until the salmon is just cooked, Serve with basil pesto-coated baby potatoes.

Benefits: Tomatoes are rich in antioxidants, which help protect against sunburn and cancer. Salmon is a good source of essential fat to help keep your skin supple.

Day 2:
BREAKFAST
Coconut Bircher muesli with mango

Mix 25 ml (1½ tbsp) coconut milk with 40 g (1½ oz) rolled oats, leave to soak and serve with 2 tbsp low-fat live natural yogurt, lime juice and 50 g (2 oz) fresh mango.

Benefits: Oats are a good source of zinc, which helps control the production of oil in the skin. Coconut milk is rich in copper, which keeps your skin elastic and flexible.

SNACK
Nectarines with ginger and pumpkin seeds

For a delicious snack, eat 100 g (3¾ oz) sliced nectarine with some grated root ginger and a handful of pumpkin seeds.

Benefits: Raw seeds eaten like this are a good source of omega 6 essential fat. Omega 6 oils can help regulate the skin's oiliness and heal blemishes.

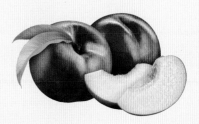

LUNCH

King prawns with coriander pesto

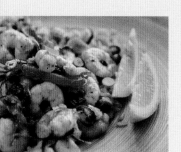

Mix pesto ingredients in a blender: 30 g (1¼ oz) cashew nuts, 10 g
(¼ oz) coriander, garlic, chilli flakes, sesame oil and some lime juice.
Serve with a wild rice salad: cook a blend of wild and brown rice
(60 g/2¼ oz uncooked), mix with spring onions (scallions), blanched
baby corn, mangetouts (snow peas), red and yellow (bell) pepper and
some soy sauce and cooked peeled prawns (shrimp).

Benefits: Shellfish are a low-fat, low-calorie source of protein and are
full of minerals, including antioxidant selenium, which can protect
your skin against ageing.

SNACK

Cashew nut and beetroot pâté

Blend some red (bell) pepper, beetroot (beets), cashew nuts and ginger
with soy sauce and cider vinegar. Serve with some fresh raw sugar
snap peas.

Benefits: Beetroot is a good source of fibre and is rich in antioxidants
which help boost the immune system. It helps build collagen to keep
your cells supple.

DINNER

Marinated beef chilli with green papaya and Asian coleslaw salad

Combine 100 g (3¾ oz) unripe green papaya, 1 tsp each of green chilli,
fresh mint and coriander (cilantro) and lemon juice with 50 g (2 oz)
each of thinly sliced red and white cabbage. Pepper 100 g (3¾ oz)
rump steak and cook in oil. Slice thinly and serve with the papaya
coleslaw and some rice noodles.

Benefits: Cabbage contains antioxidant vitamins A and C, which
help prevent sun damage.

Day 3:
BREAKFAST
Smoked salmon and scrambled egg

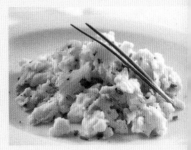

Prepare 50 g (2 oz) smoked salmon with one free-range scrambled egg, Serve with roasted baby plum tomatoes, a squeeze of lemon juice and a sprinkle of black pepper.

Benefits: The protein and retinal found in eggs helps collagen production and aids skin regeneration.

SNACK
Cherries and hazelnuts

For a delicious morning snack, eat 100 g (3¾ oz) seasonal fresh cherries with a small handful of hazelnuts.

Benefits: Cherries are a good source of vitamin C, which will help protect the skin from free-radical damage.

LUNCH
Roast chicken superfood salad

Mix salad ingredients: 40 g (1½ oz) quinoa, 15 g (½ oz) alfalfa sprouts, 30 g (1¼ oz) watercress, 30 g (1¼ oz) mangetouts (snow peas) and 80 g (3¼ oz) broccoli. Thinly slice 80 g (3¼ oz) skinless roast chicken and 80 g (3¼ oz) roast baby beetroot (beets) on top. Drizzle with lime juice.

Benefits: This salad is packed with super ingredients for the skin. Quinoa is a rich source of perfect protein and is easily digested, so it doesn't cause bloating.

SNACK
Sun-dried tomato hummus with sugar snap peas

Blend chickpeas, tahini, garlic and sun-dried tomatoes. Serve with 100 g (3¾ oz) washed, raw sugar snap peas and dip into the sun-dried tomato hummus for a healthy snack.

Benefits: Tomatoes are rich in vitamins A and C and lycopene, an important antioxidant which helps defend your skin from free-radical damage.

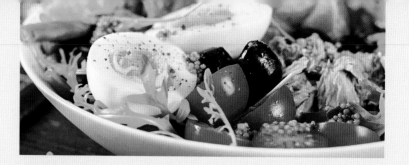

DINNER
Barbecued tuna steak niçoise

Combine 100 g (3¾ oz) green beans, 10 g (¼ oz) black olives, two ripe tomatoes, two anchovy fillets, 25 g (1 oz) hard-boiled quail eggs, seasonal salad leaves and 2 tbsp extra virgin olive oil. Mix with a red wine and Dijon mustard dressing. Chargrill a red pepper, remove the skin and slice. Barbecue 100 g (3¾ oz) yellow fin tuna steak and place on top of the salad.

Benefits: Tuna's omega 3 essential fat content helps your skin's cell walls retain moisture, preventing dry skin.

Day 4:
BREAKFAST
Fresh blackberries, cinnamon spiced apples and yogurt

Peel and roast one apple with cinnamon (180°C/gas mark 4) for 10 minutes, cool and mix it with organic, probiotic natural yogurt, berries and cashew nuts.

Benefits: Cinnamon aids blood sugar control, helping to prevent unhealthy snacking.

SNACK
Baba ghanoush with crudités

Sauté aubergine (eggplant) cubes until soft in a little olive oil. Transfer them to a food processor and combine with half a clove of garlic, 1 tsp cumin, a drizzle of lemon juice and some fresh basil leaves. Serve with 50 g (2 oz) raw carrot and 50 g (2 oz) cucumber batons.

Benefits: Aubergines are a rich source of bioflavonoids – antioxidants that protect against ageing.

LUNCH
Smoked mackerel salad with horseradish dressing

Flake a fillet of naturally smoked mackerel over a salad of mixed leaves, sliced (bell) peppers and halved cherry tomatoes. Combine the horseradish sauce with natural yogurt and drizzle over the salad.

Benefits: Mackerel is a good source of vitamin E, which has excellent moisturizing properties.

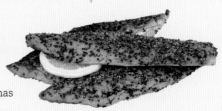

SNACK
Citrus fruit salad with dried apricots and seeds

Mix together segments of 50 g (2 oz) each of fresh orange and grapefruit with 20 g (¾ oz) chopped organic dried apricots and a small handful of black sesame seeds sprinkled on top.

Benefits: Citrus fruits are a source of antioxidants, which help build collagen to keep your cells elastic.

DINNER
Stuffed red pepper with goat's cheese

Roast half a red (bell) pepper in a pre-heated oven (180°C/gas mark 4) on the middle shelf for 10 minutes. Quarter a tomato and stuff into the pepper with a sliced garlic clove. Roast for 10 minutes. Place a slice of goat's cheese on top and grill on a high heat until bubbling. Serve with sautéed spinach, leafy greens or steamed green beans.

Benefit: Cheese is rich in vitamin A, which helps to maintain good skin health.

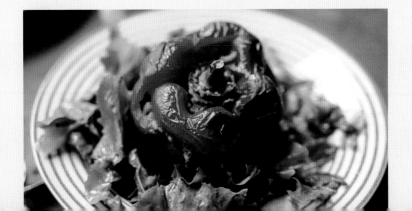

Day 5:

BREAKFAST

Watercress and cherry tomato omelette

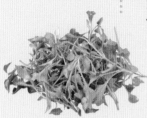

Dry fry a few halved cherry tomatoes, drizzle with olive oil and add one beaten free-range egg loosened with a little milk or water. Add a handful of fresh watercress leaves and finish under the grill.

Benefits: Watercress is full of the antioxidant beta carotene – vital for protecting against ageing.

SNACK

Bunch of fresh grapes with a small handful of Brazil nuts

Benefits: Grapes are powerful detoxifiers and can improve the condition of your skin.

LUNCH

Tiger prawns served with an orange and mint salsa

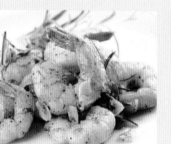

Stir fry 80 g (3¼ oz) prawns (shrimp) and cook 40 g (1½ oz) brown rice. Mix the rice with chopped coriander (cilantro) and serve on a bed of rocket (arugula) with 50 g (2 oz) kidney beans and a salsa made from blended apple, orange, ginger and mint.

Benefits: Prawns are a good source of zinc, which is needed to make collagen and elastin in your skin.

SNACK

Spiced poached pears

Lightly poach a chopped pear in water with ½ tsp Chinese five-spice and star anise. When tender, take out and serve with Greek yogurt.

Benefits: Live natural yogurt will help provide the gut with friendly bacteria to aid digestion.

DINNER

Balsamic rainbow trout

Pre-heat an oven to 180°C/gas mark 4. Place a fillet of trout on a sheet of foil, drizzle 1 tbsp balsamic vinegar over it and place a couple of

basil leaves on top. Fold up the foil to make an envelope. Place on a
baking sheet and roast for 8 minutes until the trout is just cooked.
Serve with flaked almonds, asparagus and roasted cherry tomatoes.
Benefits: Oily fish (such as trout) is a good source of essential fat,
which helps to keep cells hydrated.

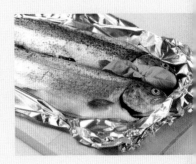

Day 6:
BREAKFAST
Strawberry and banana Bircher muesli

Blend 40 g (1½ oz) each of strawberries and bananas with 120 g (4 oz)
live natural yogurt. Stir in 30 g (1¼ oz) oats and leave for 30 minutes.
Serve with a couple of nuts on top.
Benefits: Strawberries contain alpha hydroxy acids (AHAs), which can
help to clear up blemishes.

SNACK
Avocado guacamole

Blend half an avocado with some lime juice, chilli and 1 tsp chopped
red onion. Add in half a chopped tomato. Serve with two brown
rice cakes or some corn chips.
Benefits: Avocados are a good source of vitamin E, which has
excellent moisturizing properties. Eating vegetables raw like this
means you receive their maximum nutrient content.

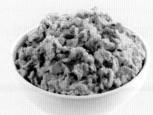

LUNCH
Roasted vegetable and buffalo mozzarella salad

Roast a selection of vegetables (red onion, courgette/zucchini, red
(bell) peppers and aubergine/eggplant) in the middle of a pre-heated
oven (200°C, gas mark 6). Steam 80 g (3¼ oz) baby potatoes and
mix with the roasted vegetables, then top with pieces of buffalo
mozzarella cheese (40 g/1½ oz). Serve on a bed of rocket (arugula)
leaves with some balsamic vinegar.
Benefits: Red peppers are a rich source of beta carotene and
vitamin C.

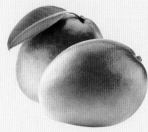

SNACK
Mango and pumpkin seeds

Serve 100 g (3¾ oz) mango with some raw pumpkin seeds.

Benefits: Mangoes are rich in vitamin C and beta carotene, and are said to cleanse the blood. Seeds are a source of omega 6 essential fat, which can help blemishes.

DINNER
Fillet of beef and shiitake noodles

Sear a small fillet of steak on a griddle and rest. Slice shiitake mushrooms and sauté them lightly in a little soy sauce. Place thin rice noodles in a bowl and pour over boiling water. Leave until cooked. Serve the noodles on a bed of rocket (arugula), topped with the thinly sliced fillet steak, mushrooms and some chopped cashew nuts, chilli and coriander (cilantro).

Benefits: Mushrooms have immune-boosting and antioxidant properties and can reduce inflammation, helping your skin to look healthier.

Day 7:
BREAKFAST
Grapefruit, rye bread and nut spread

Toast a couple of slices of rye bread. Thinly smooth a natural nut spread on top (we like Carley's Organic Rainforest Nut Butter), and serve with 100 g (3¾ oz) grapefruit pieces.

Benefits: Rye is a useful source of fibre, needed to maintain a healthy liver, which helps your skin.

SNACK
Kiwi and black sesame seeds

Peel and slice two kiwi fruit and serve with a sprinkling of black sesame seeds.

Benefits: Kiwi fruit are a rich source of vitamin C.

LUNCH
Tabbouleh salad with grilled chicken

Drizzle a free-range chicken breast in lemon juice, season with black pepper and grill until cooked through. Leave to rest. Wash half a cup of barley couscous, add half a cup of boiling water, cover and leave for 10 minutes. Cool slightly, mix with 1½ cups chopped parsley, chopped tomatoes, (bell) peppers, cucumber, the juice of half a lemon and some olive oil. Slice the chicken and serve.

Benefits: Barley couscous is an excellent source of iron and rich in minerals. Parsley is a powerful diuretic.

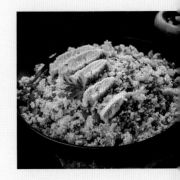

SNACK
Hot tomato salsa with crudités

Sauté a handful of halved cherry tomatoes until softened. Cool. Blend with lime juice and fresh coriander (cilantro) until mixed but still chunky. Add red chilli to the mixture, if desired. Serve with celery and sugar snap peas.

Benefits: Tomatoes are a rich source of the antioxidant lycopene and vitamin E, which protects your skin cells from ultraviolet light and free-radical damage.

DINNER
Butternut squash stuffed with feta cheese and pumpkin seeds

Halve a small butternut squash and scoop out the seeds and stringy bits. Place in a pre-heated oven (200°C/gas mark 6) on a baking sheet for 30 minutes. Sauté an onion until soft, mix with a few sun-dried tomatoes, feta cheese, pumpkin seeds and basil. Place the mix into the centre of the cooked butternut. Place in the oven for 10 minutes and serve with a mixed balsamic dressed salad.

Benefits: Butternut squash is rich in beta carotene, which helps fight signs of ageing.

STAY-YOUNG RECIPES

Look and feel your best with these anti-ageing recipes.

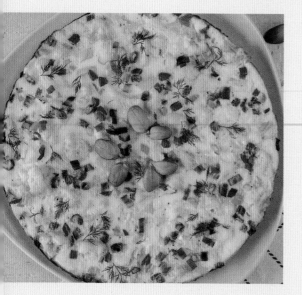

Marinated tofu and pomegranate salad (serves 2, or 4 as a starter)
Full of anti-ageing antioxidants, this salad is quick to make and is an
ideal lunch or starter.

Preparation time: 10 minutes
Method: Add 200 g (7 oz) mixed leaves to a bowl, sprinkle with a
160 g (5¼ oz) pack of marinated tofu pieces, 100 g (3¾ oz)
pomegranate seeds and 1 tbsp pumpkin seeds.
Add the grated zest and juice of an orange and a drizzle of cold-
pressed hemp oil.

♥ Tofu is a rich source of low-fat protein and a good source of iron.
♥ Pomegranates are packed with antioxidants and high in fibre.

Sweet pepper and spring onion omelette
(serves 1)
Packed with skin-saving protein, this fast dish
makes a sustaining lunch or post-gym supper.

Preparation time: 5 minutes
Cooking time: 7–10 minutes
Method: Add a quarter red (bell) pepper and a
quarter yellow pepper to a small non-stick pan
with a dash of sunflower oil.
Cook for 2–3 minutes to soften, add three
chopped spring onions (scallions), and then
cook for a further 2 minutes.
Break two eggs into another bowl and mix
with a fork but don't beat too much.

Add a further dash of oil to the pan, then add the eggs and cook for 1 minute, mixing with a fork two to three times.

Sprinkle with a tablespoon of grated mature cheddar, top with the onions and peppers, season, then fold the omelette in half with a spatula. Cook for a further minute, then turn it on to a plate and serve.

♥ Eggs are one of the only sources of vitamin D, which is essential for bone health.

Sesame-crusted salmon (serves 2)

Rich in proteins and omega 3s – the perfect beauty beauty foods – this salmon supper is a facelift on a plate!

Preparation time: 10 minutes

Cooking time: 15 minutes

Method: Coat two salmon steaks with the juice of half a lemon out on a plate and sprinkle with 2 tbsp sesame seeds, making sure they're well coated. Place on a lightly oiled baking sheet, sprinkle any remaining seeds on top and bake in a pre-heated at 180°C/gas mark 4 for 12–15 minutes.

While the salmon cooks, add a 300 g (11 oz) bag of stir-fry vegetables (try one with soya beans) to a pan with a dash of toasted sesame oil and cook for 3–5 minutes over a high heat.

Place the vegetables on a dish, break the salmon into chunks and arrange on top, then drizzle with 1 tsp soy sauce and a squeeze of lemon juice.

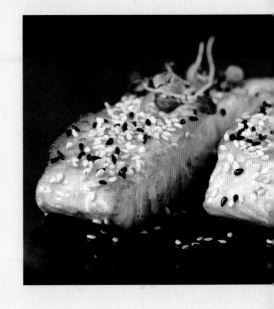

♥ Salmon is an excellent form of protein, low in saturated fat and high in omega 3 and vitamin D.

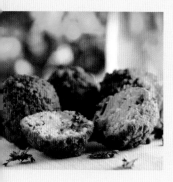

Falafel sprouted seed and tahini wrap (serves 1)

Packed with vitamins, this quick and easy lunch is the perfect nutrient boost when you're on the run.

Preparation time: 5 minutes

Method: Spread 1 tbsp low-fat cottage cheese on a wholemeal tortilla and add a handful of sprouts (try alfalfa, radish and sunflower sprouts).

Add two to three crumbled falafels and drizzle with 2 tbsp tahini. Roll it up and enjoy!

♥ Chickpeas boost digestive and heart health, and are a good source of folate.

Quinoa, sunflower seed and apricot pilaf (serves 4)

This pilaf makes and excellent side dish and is also ideal to take to work for lunch.

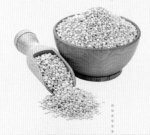

Preparation time: 10 minutes

Cooking time: 20 minutes

Method: Add a dash of sunflower oil to a pan with a finely chopped onion and stir regularly for 3 minutes.

Add a chopped leek, 2 heaped tsp ground cumin, 1 level tsp chilli flakes and a good pinch of salt, 175 g (6 oz) quinoa and 500 ml (2 cups) boiling water and simmer gently for 15 minutes.

Meanwhile, chop 75 g (3 oz) dried apricots and mix with 2 tbsp sunflower seeds and 50 g (2 oz) chopped coriander (cilantro), the juice and grated zest of an unwaxed lemon and 1 tbsp extra virgin olive oil. When the quinoa is cooked, fluff it up with a fork and mix with the apricot mixture.

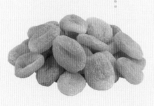

♥ Dried apricots are a good source of iron, which builds red blood cells, and potassium, which aids muscle function.

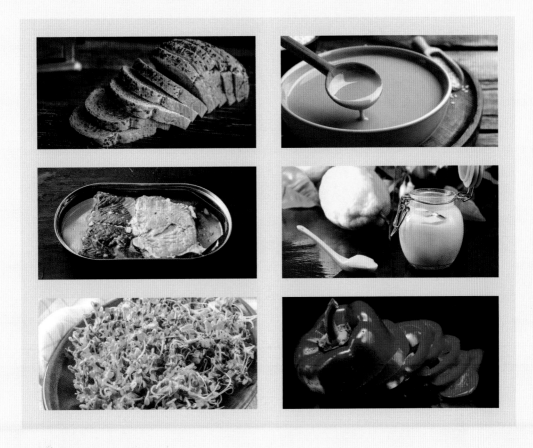

Superfood sandwich (serves 2)

A few nutrient-packed ingredients can turn an ordinary sandwich
into a power-packed lunch.

Preparation time: 10 minutes

Method: Spread four slices of wholegrain seeded bread with
1 tbsp tahini.

Mix a 213 g (7 oz) can of sockeye salmon with the juice of half a lemon,
1 tbsp live natural yogurt and some black pepper.

Divide the salmon, 75 g (3 oz) alfalfa and radish sprouts, and half a
thinly sliced red pepper to make two sandwiches.

YOUR FITNESS

Regular exercise is vital to defend your body against ageing. It protects your major organs, gives you energy and helps you maintain a healthy weight. It is also lowers the risk of diseases such as dementia, osteoporosis and diabetes. In this chapter, learn how to hold back the years with our age-busting workouts.

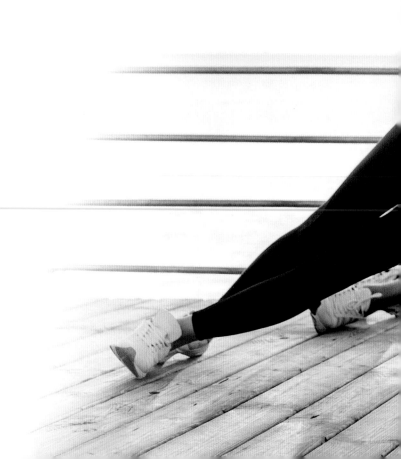

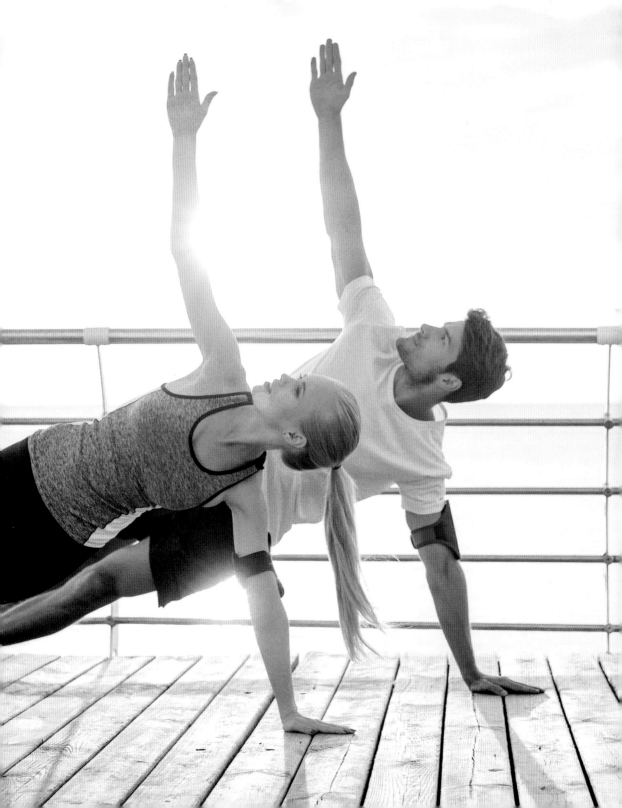

AGE-FIGHTING FIT

Regular exercise won't just keep you toned and energized – the latest research shows it keeps your body young too.

There's nothing more youthful than the radiant glow you get after exercising. And research shows that staying active has anti-ageing benefits from top to toe.

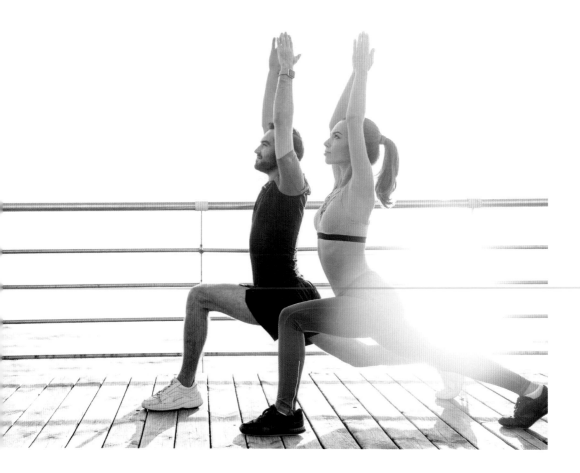

IT AGE-PROOFS YOUR CELLS

Exercise keeps you young from the inside out. A study at Saarland University in Germany found that exercise hinders the shortening of telomeres – the protective caps on the ends of all our chromosomes. Telomeres are similar to the plastic tips on the end of shoelaces that stop them unravelling. As telomeres shorten, a cell becomes more susceptible to dying. The researchers also suggested a sedentary lifestyle can make you more susceptible to free-radical damage and inflammation at a cellular level.

IT PROTECTS YOUR HEART

Exercise has rich and multi-layered benefits for your heart, lowering body fat, blood pressure and risk of diabetes, as well as raising levels of heart-protective high-density lipoprotein (HDL) cholesterol.

IT'S DE-STRESSING

Experts at the University of Missouri, Columbia in the US have found relatively high-intensity exercise is one of the best tools we have for reducing stress and anxiety. And all the better if you exercise outdoors – a study at the University of Essex showed that a five-minute burst of outdoor activity will lift your mood.

IT HELPS AGE-ERASE YOUR SKIN

When you exercise, you increase your circulation and get the blood flowing around your body so that it brings nutrients and oxygen to your skin – and a wonderful rosy glow.

IT BOOSTS YOUR BRAIN CELLS

Countless studies show that regular exercise, such as running, can help create new brain cells. It can also significantly lower your risk of age-related brain decline and dementia.

DON'T OVERDO IT!

Over-exercising can be just as ageing as doing no activity. It puts you at risk of injury, can reduce your body fat levels enough to risk your fertility and bone health, stress your joints and cause cellular inflammation. And if you're a fan of working out outside, you're likely to expose yourself to greater levels of sun damage – so wear UV protection.

US research also shows that the loss of skin plumpness that comes with being underweight is ageing. A study at Case Western Reserve University in Cleveland, Ohio showed a link between weight and our predicted age. They found people with a low BMI are perceived to be older than they are.

YOUR EXERCISE PRESCRIPTION

Your anti-ageing workout programme should include:

Cardiovascular activity

Aerobic exercise, such as dancing and swimming, boosts your circulation, heart and lungs. Make sure some of your sessions are weight-bearing, such as walking and running, to give your bones a workout. If you have joint problems, brisk walking will suffice.

Resistance training

Weight training helps to build muscle and fire your metabolism. It also strengthens your bones and can improve your flexibility and co-ordination.

Stretching

Flexibility exercises such as Pilates and yoga build strength in your joints and muscles, and are proven to reduce stress.

Mental training

Any physical activity that gets you interacting with others, taxes your brain with complicated rules or tests your memory is fantastic for keeping your brain healthy and young. Think dancing, orienteering or tennis.

IT CUTS YOUR CANCER RISK

Regular exercise can slash women's risk of breast cancer, confirms a study of 74,000 women at the Fred Hutchinson Cancer Research Center in Seattle. And a US review of 52 studies found it can cut the risk of colon cancer by up to 24 per cent.

IT KEEPS YOUR BONES YOUNG

Many factors contribute to bone density, but physical activity is one of the most powerful and proactive ways of maintaining a healthy bone mass. The best bone-stimulating activity is weight-bearing exercise, such as running, walking and weight training. Keeping fit can also help you avoid the loss of flexibility that tends to come with age.

IT BALANCES YOUR HORMONES

As well as helping minimize women's PMS symptoms, a study published in the journal *Medicine & Science in Sports & Exercise* shows that if you remain active up to and during the menopause, you can ease common symptoms including anxiety, depression and stress.

IT'S NEVER TOO LATE ...

Regular exercising is essential from a young age, but it's such a powerful anti-ageing weapon that you'll still get the benefits if you start later. A study by Boston's Brigham and Women's Hospital in the US showed that even taking up exercise after the age of 70, along with eating healthily and not smoking, can boost your life expectancy by 50 per cent.

YOUR METABOLISM

Have you found it harder to lose weight or keep it off as you've got older? Diet, exercise and regular strength training can all help.

Some people think our metabolic rate naturally slows down as we get older, but in fact it's more due to the fact that our bodies lose lean muscle mass as we age. Muscle is metabolically active, so the less lean muscle tissue you have, the less efficient your body. You can offset the process of losing lean muscle tissue with regular strength training, either by doing a Body Pump class or using weights at the gym. Kettlebell classes are also good for improving strength, as well as shaping and toning your body. But if you've noticed the pounds have been creeping on a bit in the past few years, it's important to stress that exercise alone won't make you slim. In fact, diet is more important than exercise when it comes to losing weight. While being regularly active will burn calories and help you stay in shape, you simply can't out-exercise a bad diet.

In fact, some nutritional experts claim that weight loss is generally 75 per cent diet and 25 per cent exercise. When you think about it, this makes sense. If you were to run for 30 minutes, you would burn off approximately 300 calories. You could put most of those calories back into your body quite quickly just

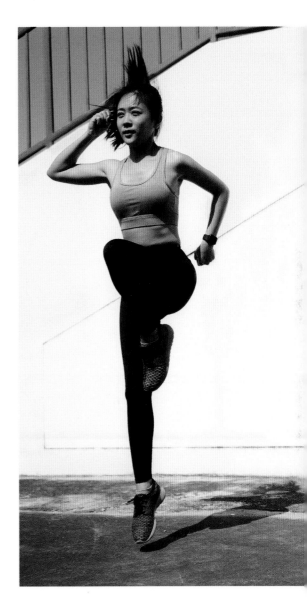

BEST WAYS TO BOOST YOUR METABOLISM

Do regular aerobic exercise – Aim to do around 150 minutes per week of activities such as walking, cycling, going to the gym, swimming, running, jogging or classes like circuit training, all of which work you at a fast pace.

Do strength training – Increase your ratio of lean muscle tissue and the results will speak for

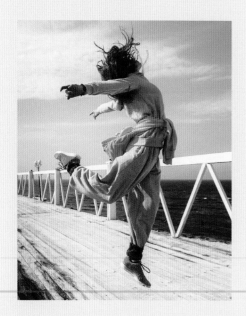

themselves. Not only will you be more toned, but you will have more lean muscle, which is more metabolically active.

Do high-intensity interval training (HIIT) – This means working hard for set intervals (such as for one minute), then doing a slower pace for a minute to recover, then repeating. You can do HIIT training on any cardio machine in the gym.

Stay on the move – Try to stay as active as you can during the day. Move around. Have meetings where you walk around rather than sit at a desk, if possible. Being constantly active will make a difference to your metabolic rate. Walking the kids to school, taking a walk at lunchtime or cycling to the station instead of driving will all add up.

Drink coffee (in moderation) – Caffeine can help to increase your metabolic rate, but make sure you don't drink too much, as it can increase your stress levels. Caffeine can kick-start a process called lipolysis, which is when your body starts to break down fat stores for energy. Experts debate how effective it is, but it is used in many weight-loss supplements.

by consuming a large chocolate bar or by eating about four biscuits. It's very easy to put the calories back on quickly, but it takes considerably longer to burn them off.

While exercise will support your weight loss, it isn't the most important component. The best way to strip fat and boost your metabolism is to combine your exercise routine with a healthy diet.

WONDER WORKOUTS

We've cherry-picked the most effective forms of exercise to help you keep those tell-tale signs of ageing at bay.

All exercise is anti-ageing, but choose carefully and you can target the areas of your health and body that you are most concerned about to stay fit and youthful. From your bones and heart to your pelvic floor, every workout has different benefits.

WALKING

Accessible, thrifty and a super-effective exercise, regular walking is linked to a lower risk of heart disease, diabetes, high blood pressure and osteoporosis. But don't dawdle – experts believe that your speed might help you monitor how healthy you are. A study at the University of Pittsburgh in the US found that a person with a walking speed slower than 0.6 m (2 ft) per second may be at increased risk of poor health.

RUNNING

As well as being good for your heart, running is also a form of weight-bearing exercise, meaning it challenges and strengthens your skeleton. A 21-year study at Stanford University in the US showed that runners have fewer disabilities, stay active for longer and halve their risk of an early death.

YOGA

Yoga is a true mind-body experience. It offers a resistance workout, enhancing muscle strength and flexibility, and can help offset lower back pain, stiff joints and loss of balance. But yoga is also an effective stress reliever – in an analysis of its effect on the brain chemical GABA, researchers from Boston University School of Medicine in the US found it's superior to other exercise in terms of its positive effect on mood and anxiety.

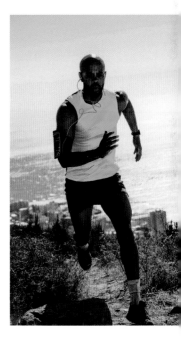

Researchers have found that hitting the dance floor helps you ward off dementia.

PILATES

Pilates strengthens the core muscles that protect your spine – but it also enhances joint flexibility, balance and coordination. Crucially, it's great for injury rehabilitation and is gentle enough to be continued into old age. According to a study of 60 women over the age of 65 published in the *Journal of Sports Science and Medicine*, a sustained programme can enhance mobility.

DANCING

Dancing is a weight-bearing form of aerobic exercise and can rev up your grey matter too. Researchers at Albert Einstein College of Medicine in New York found that alongside playing musical instruments, reading and playing board games, hitting the dance floor helps you ward off dementia. Try high-octane Zumba if ballroom is too sedate for you!

SWIMMING

An excellent aerobic workout, great for muscle tone and joint mobility, swimming is kind on an ageing body as your weight is fully supported. Research at Indiana University in the US found that regular and moderately intensive swimming can halt the downward decline of your key age markers, blood pressure, muscle mass, blood chemistry and pulmonary function.

PELVIC FLOOR EXERCISES

It's said that around four million British women have stress incontinence. This occurs when the sphincter muscle isn't strong enough to withstand bladder pressure, and is common after childbirth and pregnancy. One preventative step is to shape up your pelvic floor muscles, which wrap from the front of your pelvis to your tail bone and keep all your internal organs in place. Daily Kegel exercises are a must. Sit on the arm of a chair with your legs slightly apart then contract your muscles around your urethra, vagina and rectum as if trying to stop yourself peeing. Don't strain, hold, then relax. Do 10 reps of 10 seconds every day.

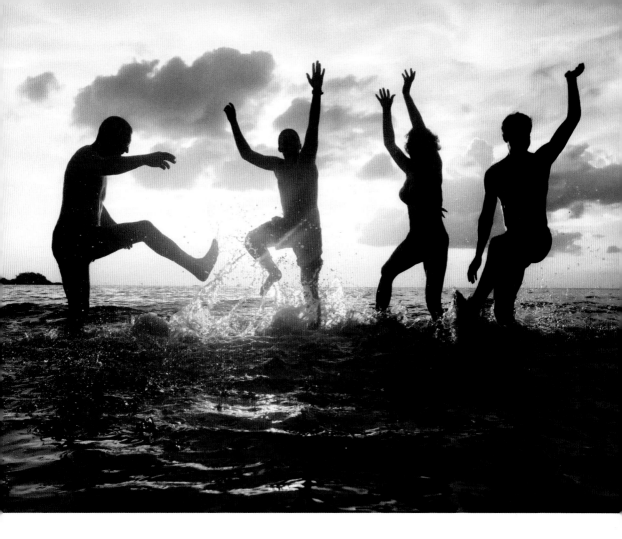

RESISTANCE TRAINING

Working with dumbbells or weighted kit, such as kettlebells, is something we should all prioritize throughout our lives. Various age-related conditions – including osteoporosis, joint immobility and, crucially, dramatic muscle loss (sarcopenia) – can be prevented or at least slowed by strengthening your muscles with resistance work. And it's never too late to start weight training. A study at the Buck Institute for Age Research in California found it has the potential to actually reverse muscle ageing because it improves the way our muscle cells work.

ACT YOUR AGE

Tailor your exercise programme to suit your age, and keep
your youthful glow.

In our childhood it was leapfrog, in our teens, cross country or athletics.
But too often, as we reach adulthood, our activity levels decline – just
when our bodies really need exercise. While high-impact aerobics or
running may not be your thing, there's always a workout that's just right
for you and your body's needs. From bone-building resistance workouts
to rejuvenating yoga, finding the right workout for your age can help you
stay fit, strong and slim through the years.

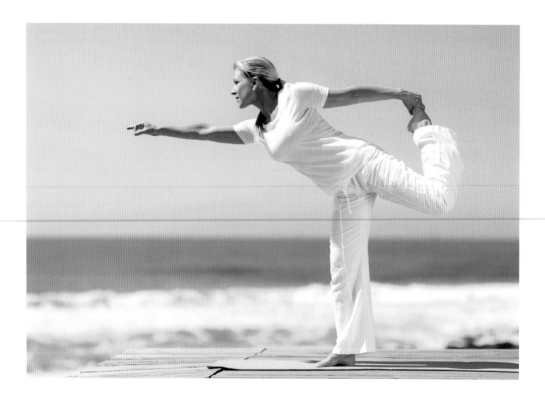

IN YOUR 20s

Time to build your cardio health and bone strength. You're at the peak of your fitness in your 20s, and as your body is still building up bone mass, maximize your reserves by working out regularly, especially with weight-bearing exercise. Although the body's natural drop in aerobic fitness (10 per cent a decade) starts in your 20s, you can cut this by as much as 50 per cent by exercising. It's likely you'll be bursting with natural energy, but if you find it hard to motivate yourself, try group or competitive sports, such as basketball, tennis and hockey, or something upbeat such as dancing, so you can feed off the enthusiasm of others. Studies also show that exercise will also help women manage PMS-related symptoms including mood swings and abdominal cramps. Boosting your lean muscle mass will increase your metabolism and help you burn off calories.

IN YOUR 30s

Your 30s are often very demanding, with work and family needs vying for your attention. Staying fit will help you cope with this busy decade as well as ward of the health challenges of the next. Now's the time to ratchet up your resistance exercise. This will help you defy the natural decline in muscle, boosting your metabolic rate and helping keep your weight in check. Remember your muscles adapt quickly, so ramp up your programme every six to eight weeks by using heavier weights or increasing your reps. Age-related muscle loss is greater in your lower body than your upper, so make sure your programmes are balanced. Pregnancy and long-term habits such as working in an office or carrying a heavy bag can have an impact on your back and flexibility, so make time for a weekly Pilates or yoga class. If your work and family commitments mean you're squeezed for time, try high-impact short circuits, start active commuting by walking or cycling to work, or explore home workouts.

IN YOUR 40s

Prevent middle-age spread with high-impact and endurance workouts. Just because you've hit the big four-O, it doesn't mean your fitness will decline. Simply carry on looking after your body and keep challenging yourself.

Adapt your resistance programme regularly to increase the demand on your muscles, and ditto your aerobic programme. Studies show you can maintain your VO2 max – your aerobic capacity – with endurance training. Any activity that requires staying power will do. For a challenge, enter a long-distance running event. Besides the physical benefits, having something to focus on will fire your motivation levels, especially if you're raising funds for charity.

Or try a triathlon – the combination of running with low-impact swimming and cycling is much kinder on joints than pure running.

Prioritize weight-bearing exercise – as women approach the menopause and experience a dip in the bone-protective hormone oestrogen, this is the time to accrue some strength. But don't overdo things. Your body is less forgiving in your 40s than in your 20s, so take a steady approach to training and ask a professional for guidance if necessary.

IN YOUR 50s PLUS

Keep your heart healthy with regular aerobic exercise – but be kind to yourself! Don't be misled into thinking it's all downhill from here. More than half a million Brits over 50 have run a marathon. The key now is to be conscious of your health and fitness on a daily basis and follow a structured exercise plan to combat age-related conditions. The biggie for women this decade is the menopause, so take action to prevent deep visceral fat from settling around your waistline. It can narrow your arteries and raise cholesterol, and increase your risk of type 2 diabetes, high blood pressure and dementia. It's also a risk factor for breast and colon cancers.

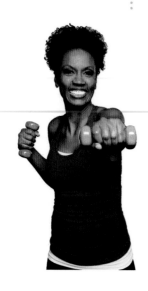

But tummy fat is not inevitable. Reduce fat levels all over with a sustained aerobic and resistance programme. If you're worried about your joints, focus on low-impact aerobic exercise such as walking, cycling and swimming. Using a step is particularly good – it combines cardio and strength exercise but, because you're moving against gravity, pressure on your joints is minimized. To lift your mood and ease stress, try a sociable form of exercise, such as dancing. Or try t'ai chi – it's great for balance, coordination, building bone mass and, according to researchers at the University of California, Los Angeles, can ease depression.

ANTI-AGEING WORKOUT

Tone up your trouble zones and watch the years melt away with this age-defying exercise plan.

The following workout has been devised to help you banish bingo wings and muffin tops for good — all those stubborn areas that stop you feeling svelte and youthful. The exercises have the added benefit of being weight-bearing, so they'll also help boost your bone density. To get maximum benefits, add impact exercises, such as walking, running or aerobics where both feet are not in contact with the floor at the same time. Run to boost both your bone density and energy, or use a step to get a high-impact workout.

BEFORE YOU BEGIN...

This quick plan only takes 30 minutes, providing you practise it three times a week. For better results, gradually make the workout more intense by adding more weight, extra reps or both, week by week. If you do your cardio before the exercises, your performance will be significantly better, as your muscles will be warm, making you more flexible.

LOOK THE PART

To safeguard your wellbeing, wear the right gear — that means a supportive bra, sports-specific socks, good trainers, sweat-wicking tee and snug capri pants, shorts or leggings.

GET KITTED UP

If you're working out at home, buying some essential kit can elevate your workout to a new level. Aside from an exercise mat, think about

Wear a supportive bra, good trainers and a sweat-wicking tee when you work out.

YOUR WORKOUT ESSENTIALS

All you need are a few props to exercise at home:

- Tone up all over with an exercise band.
- Add challenge with a set of dumbbells.
- Stay comfortable with an exercise mat.

getting a set of dumbbells, ankle and wrist weights, a gym ball – the added wobble will engage your stabilizing muscles – and a Dyna-Band or similar resistance band.

STAY SAFE

Always warm up to prepare your muscles and joints, and engage your core muscles to protect your back. Perform each exercise with precision, but don't get carried away. Don't exercise if you're unwell, stop immediately if you feel pain, and progress your workouts incrementally. Post workout, elongate your muscles and flush out lactic acid to prevent soreness by stretching for at least five minutes.

Blast bingo wings

Benefits: This exercise will work the back of your arms. Women have a tendency to carry fat here, and unless you work it regularly, the skin can become saggy.

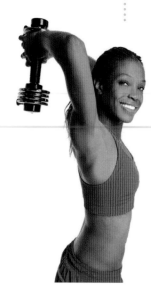

- Start with a strong posture, a weight in each hand. Take your legs wider than shoulder-width apart and bend your knees slightly to remove any tension from your lower back. Tilt your pelvis forward and keep your stomach engaged.
- Raise your hands above your head, bringing your upper arms up close to your ears.
  - Bend your arms from the elbows, taking the weights behind your head. For maximum results, keep your upper arms still and pressed close to your ears. Keep doing this exercise until you can't do any more, then repeat with one weight only.
    - Once you've exhausted your arms using one weight, repeat the exercise using your body weight only, pressing your palms together to create tension in the arms. Repeat on the other side.

Reps: As many as you can.

Total body toner

Benefits: This exercise works your legs, bottom and chest. It helps co-ordination, control and building awareness of your core.

- Start by lunging forwards on one leg, making sure your front knee doesn't extend beyond your toes.
- Hold a weight in each hand, palms facing in, and pull in your abdominal muscles. Raise your arms in front of you, elbows bent, to chest height.
- As you exhale, extend your back leg off the ground without arching your lower back. Straighten your arms and raise them in front of you to head height. Repeat on the other side.

Reps: Beginners 10 on each side; intermediates 20; advanced 30.

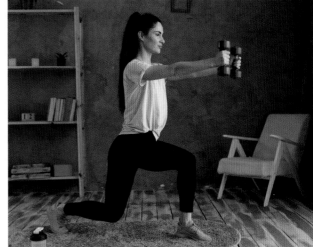

Hip toner

Benefits: This is a great move for working and toning your outer thighs and hips – it really hits the spot.

- Lie on your right side and bend your hips and knees to 90-degree angles. Rest your head in the palm of your right hand and bring the other hand to the floor in front of your chest for support. Extend your upper leg, bending 90 degrees at the hip. Flex the upper foot and point the toes towards the floor, heel towards the ceiling.
- Exhale and lift your leg up and down, keeping your stomach engaged. Don't roll backwards as you raise your leg; just lift your leg slightly above the height of your hips. Repeat to the other side.

Reps: Beginners 20 each side; intermediates 30 for two sets; advanced 30 for three sets, or two sets using ankle weights.

Firm your thighs

Benefits: Tones up your inner thighs.

- Lie on your right side, resting your head on your right hand. Bend your left leg and place the foot on the ground in front of your right thigh. With your left arm, reach through to grab your left ankle.
- Keep your body in a straight line, in contact with the ground. Move your right leg up, exhaling as you do so, with it fully extended. Flex your foot. Keep your right leg in line with the rest of your body and don't touch the ground as you lower it. Repeat on the other side.

Reps: Beginners 20 each side; intermediates 20 each side for two sets; advanced 30 each side for three sets, or two sets with ankle weights.

Boost your chest

Benefits: This is a great stabilizer for activating your core and working your chest muscles.

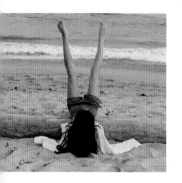

- Lying on your back, bring both legs straight up in the air. Draw your navel to your spine and press your lower back into the floor. Flex your feet and keep your legs straight. Raise your arms so your hands are straight above your shoulders. Take your arms out to the sides, with your elbows slightly bent. Return to the start position.
- Advanced version: Extend your legs further away from your body to increase the challenge to your core muscles. Taking one arm to the floor, slightly bend the elbow, without the arm touching the floor. Repeat with the other arm.

Reps: Beginners 10 each side for two sets; intermediates and advanced 20 each side for two sets.

Tone up your bottom

Benefits: This is a great exercise for building a high, perky bottom and hopefully keeping it there. It's also a great core exercise.

- Start on all fours, toes curled under and resting on your forearms. Raise one leg, letting your heel lead the way and with the sole of your foot facing the ceiling.
- Keep your elbows under your chest and avoid leaning too far forwards.

Keep your stomach engaged and maintain a neutral spine. Lower your knee to the opposite heel, keeping the rest of the body still as you do so.
Reps: Beginners 20 each side; intermediates 20 each side for two sets; advanced 30 each side for three sets, or two sets using ankle weights.

Flatten your belly
Benefits: This is excellent for toning up your tummy muscles.

- Lying on the floor, extend your legs fully and rest your left heel on top of your right toes, keeping your ankles flexed. Press your lower back into the floor and keep your head in line with your spine. Beginners should have both hands supporting the neck. Intermediates and advanced should have one arm fully extended, while the other hand grips the upper arm to support your head. Bend your legs slightly to keep your lower back supported.
- Engage your core throughout the move, exhaling as you lift your shoulders off the mat and inhaling as you lower down. You only need a 45-degree lift for your stomach muscles to be contracted. If you come up beyond that, you engage the hip flexors and the lower back.

Reps: Beginners two sets of 20; intermediates four sets of 20; advanced three sets of as many sit-ups as you can before tiring.

Strengthen your back
Benefits: This works your side, loosening your lower back as well as toning your midriff.

- Stand with your legs wider than hip-width apart, knees slightly bent. Hook a resistance band under your right foot and grasp both ends with your right hand. Focus on your stomach muscles, pulling in your tummy and clenching your bottom.
- Place both hands on your waist and, on an out-breath, take one arm down by your side. Allow your body to follow your arm, but avoid leaning forwards. Pull back up to the starting position. Deepen the side stretch each time.

Reps: Beginners 20, both sides, for two sets; intermediates 30, both sides, for two sets; advanced 40, both sides, for two sets.

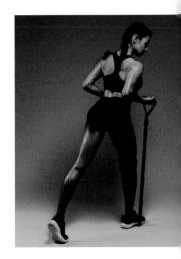

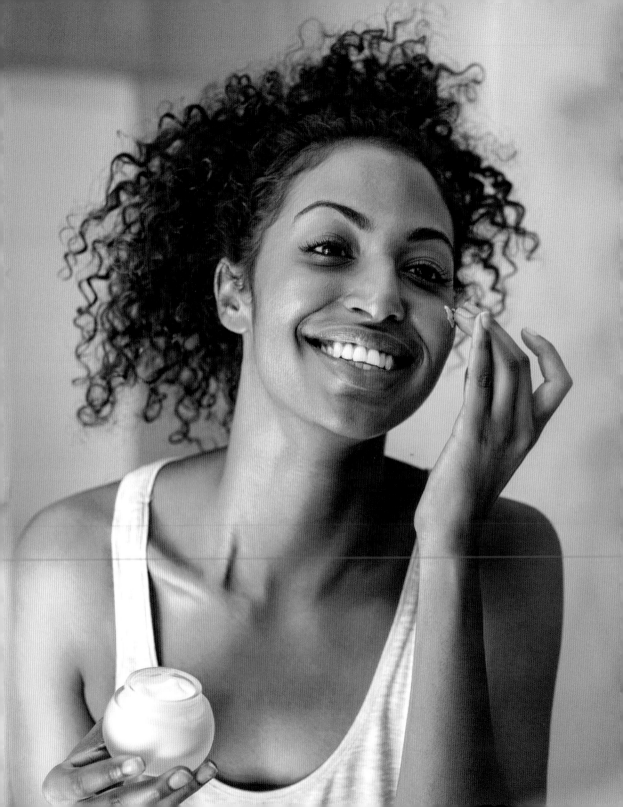

YOUR FACE

Plump and radiant skin, bright eyes, glossy hair and a sparking smile are all synonymous with youthful looks. Learn how to keep your looks in tip-top shape with our holistic approach to beauty.

DAILY RITUALS

A regular skincare routine is the basis of a radiant, healthy and youthful complexion.

Just as your body needs a regular and sustained fitness programme to stay trim and toned, your complexion demands a dedicated approach too. And irrespective of your age or skin type, the fundamentals of skincare are the same. Your skin is a complex and delicate organ, but the principles of caring for it are straightforward and common-sense.

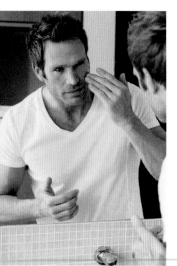

CLEANSE

A good cleanse is essential, not only to remove make-up residue, dirt and grime, but also to shift dead cells and sebum so your skin is left clearer. Apply your cleanser to dry skin, using a light, circular massage technique to bring fresh blood to the skin surface and reduce puffiness. It's tempting to go for products with a lathering quality so your face is squeaky clean, but these tend to be harsh on your skin. Try nourishing cream cleansers to keep your skin hydrated and prevent sensitivity. Soaps are most definitely out.

TONE

It's not essential, but a gentle sweep of toner across your face can help remove those last few traces of cleanser, and refresh and hydrate your skin. Give alcohol-based products the cold shoulder – it's best go for nutrient-rich products with natural skin benefits, such as aloe vera, cucumber, calendula and rosewater.

MOISTURIZE

Your skin contains a natural lipid barrier to protect it against the elements and invaders, such as pollution and dirt. By applying a moisturizer, you're enhancing the strength of your skin's innate shield and preserving the hydration levels in its deep layers. Choose a protective Sun Protection Factor (SPF) day cream and an intensive moisturizer or face oil at night. Even if you think your skin is oily, moisturizing is essential – use lighter products based on plant oils, so your complexion doesn't get congested.

A moisturizer or foundation with a broad-spectrum SPF 15 protection, even on cloudy days, will help prevent UV damage. Added antioxidants are a bonus too. And don't forget to apply to your lips and neck. Use a stronger sunscreen if you're spending lots of time outside.

EXFOLIATE

Gentle exfoliation will speed up your skin's cellular turnover, but we don't mean abrasive, grainy products – they're a bad idea for sensitive and mature skins. Using a soft muslin cloth is ideal or, for a thorough, occasional exfoliation, choose products that contain alpha hydroxy acids (AHAs) – chemical compounds found in citric fruits and cane sugar, which act as a natural exfoliant. Or pick products containing fine jojoba beads. How often you use them depends on your skin type, but start with once or twice a week. If your skin still appears dull or flaky, use more regularly.

SUPER SCIENTIFIC STUFF!

Here's a guide to the latest high-tech skincare ingredients...

AHAs and BHAs – Alpha hydroxy acids (AHAs) or fruit acids such a citric or glycolic acids, and less harsh beta hydroxy acids (BHAs) including salicylic acid, are exfoliating, brightening and can help control pigmentation and iron out roughness.

Retinol and retinyl palmate – Vitamin A is an important ant-ageing skin nutrient. These two ingredients (retinyl is better suited to sensitive skin) are topical versions of the vitamin and enhance skin radiance and condition.

Hyaluronic acid – A naturally occurring substance in your body's connective tissues that declines with age. When applied topically, it can help to plump out fine lines and beef up your skin.

Peptides – Combinations of amino acids and peptides promote collagen production and have firming properties.

Ceramides – These are lipids (fat and oil-like substances) that lock moisture into the skin.

L-ascorbic acid – A stable, topical form of vitamin C that supports collagen production.

Glycerine – This draws and locks in moisture to help hydrate the skin.

Alpha-lipoic acid – A water- and fat-soluble antioxidant that can give your skin a radiant glow.

BE BEAUTIFUL FOREVER

Your skin has different needs in each decade. If you tailor your regime accordingly, you can look fabulous whatever your age.

Your skin changes markedly through the decades, from breakouts in your 20s and fine lines in your 30s, to loss of elasticity in your 40s, and sagging and dryness in your 50s and 60s. While a consistent skincare regime is essential throughout your life, subtle tweaks can help you manage these changes. Here's how to tailor your regime accordingly and look fabulous, whatever your age.

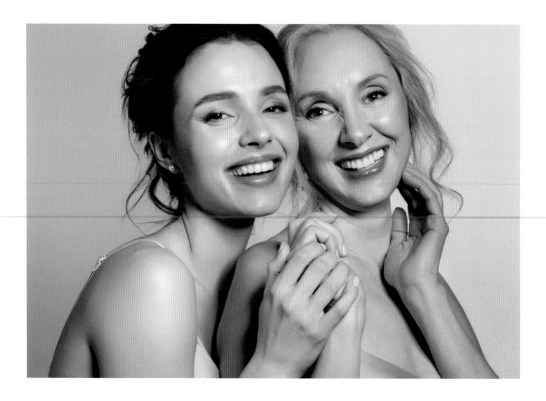

IN YOUR 20s
Establish good skincare habits

Teenage discord gives way to plumpness and luminosity in your 20s, providing you have a healthy lifestyle.

Your skin's rate of cell renewal is on your side in your 20s, so this is the time to start a dedicated cleanse, tone and moisturize routine. Always remove your make-up before you go to bed. Ideally, avoid using cleansing wipes – they leave a residue of product on your skin. Use a gentle exfoliator regularly. If your skin is still oily, use light moisturizers and oil-free make-up. Don't treat it harshly – abrasive products will strip out the natural oils and leave the upper layers of your skin dry and irritated. Your skin may still be prone to spots in your early 20s but if acne is a serious problem, see your GP and ask to be referred to a dermatologist. For skin scarred from acne, try massaging it with rosehip seed oil.

Don't drown your skin in products – invest in some quality key essentials that are based on natural ingredients.

Although your skin looks after itself, don't be complacent – damage it now and it will show later down the line. You may not see sun damage, but it could be accumulating on the sly, so use a daily moisturizer or foundation with a broad-spectrum SPF protection.

Eat plenty of antioxidant-rich fruit and vegetables to keep your skin radiant. A homemade smoothie in the morning can help you reach your five-a-day. Drink plenty of water to keep your skin hydrated, and minimize alcohol intake.

Stay young: Always use sun protection and follow a regular skincare regime to help prevent premature ageing.

IN YOUR 30s
Adapt your regime as your skin changes

A decline in collagen and elastin, along with habitual expressions, may cause fine lines to develop around your eyes, mouth and across your forehead in your 30s.

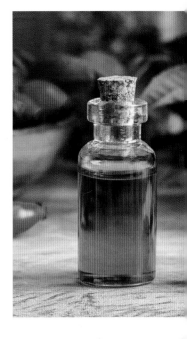

Rosehip seed oil hydrates, exfoliates and moisturizes your skin, and can also help to reduce inflammation.

The delicate skin under your eyes thins and you may experience dark circles and puffiness. Add an anti-ageing eye cream to your regime and wear sunglasses to protect against the ageing effects of UV rays. Red spider veins may also start to appear – the cheeks are particularly vulnerable – so avoid using hot water on your skin and be scrupulous about sun protection. If you have a hectic lifestyle, try to get lots of regenerative sleep and apply a vitamin-packed night cream.

Cell turnover declines and your skin will be duller than in your 20s, so use hydrating masks and gentle exfoliants regularly. Enlarged pores may be an issue, so don't overload your complexion with heavy products.

Stay young: If your skin is looking dull, use hydrating masks and gentle exfoliants regularly.

IN YOUR 40s
Protect against sun damage

Cell renewal slows down when you enter your fifth decade, so give your complexion a helping hand. Try a face cream that contains alpha hydroxy acids (AHAs) and gently exfoliate on a regular basis. Your skin will appear much brighter and more youthful as a result. Levels of your skin's natural oils (sebum) are likely to be lower now than in your 20s, so opt for creamy, hydrating products. If you had oily skin in your youth, you may find that it's more manageable now.

Because the skin's subcutaneous layer loses fat in this decade, your skin can lose some plumpness. Make sure you're getting enough essential fatty acids and phytoestrogens in your diet and look for anti-ageing products containing peptides and ceramides.

Don't spend so much time on your face that you neglect your hands and neck – they are a classic age giveaway! Cleanse, exfoliate, tone and moisturize your neck regularly, and use a moisturizing hand cream on your hands several times a day.

This is the age when you'll start to see signs of accumulated sun damage, such as age spots and crepey skin, so always wear SPF cream.

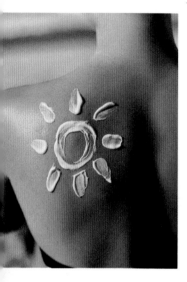

The number after the SPF of a sunscreen indicates how well it protects against sunburn. The higher the number, the more protection it gives.

Your skin will also be drier, particularly for women starting to experience the first signs of the menopause, and blemishes will take longer to heal, so invest in regular facials.

Stay young: Treat your complexion with respect, focusing on hydrating products such as luxuriant skin oils.

IN YOUR 50s PLUS
Ramp up the richness

Your skin becomes thinner, less radiant and more translucent in your 50s, and, as oestrogen levels fall in female skin and oil glands contract, it may become more sensitive. You'll also be more prone to bruising. Avoid harsh treatments and allergens, such as perfumes, drink plenty of water every day and make sure you're getting plenty of healing and moisturizing essential fatty acids in your diet.

If it's a jowly appearance that's the problem, try regular face exercises or lifting salon treatments. Treat your skin with respect and upgrade your products across the board, including your make-up, to the most emollient (moisture-locking) types.

Age spots become noticeable now, so increase your sun protection regime. You could try a salon treatment to help fade problem areas. Skin tags are common – about 50 to 60 per cent of over 50s experience them. If they're irritating you, see your GP, who can remove them fairly effortlessly.

To combat pigmentation and inflammation, avoid any foods (spices, alcohol and caffeine) that can cause flushing. Protect your skin in the elements, whether the weather is hot or cold. Switch to mineral-based make-up, redness-calming moisturizers and ask your doctor for advice if redness becomes a persistent issue.

Stay young: Avoid harsh treatments and allergens, such as perfumes, and make sure you drink plenty of water every day.

Aim to drink six to eight glasses of water a day, or more if the weather is warm.

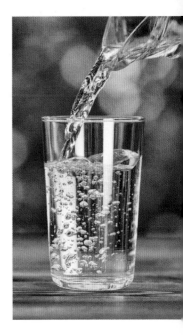

KEEP YOUR FACE FIT

Smooth away lines the natural way with this facial workout.

We all know there's no cream in the world that will instantly give us a flat stomach, firm thighs or beautiful sculpted arms. The best way to get a fit body is through exercise. But when it comes to our faces, we happily rely on creams without regard for our facial muscles.

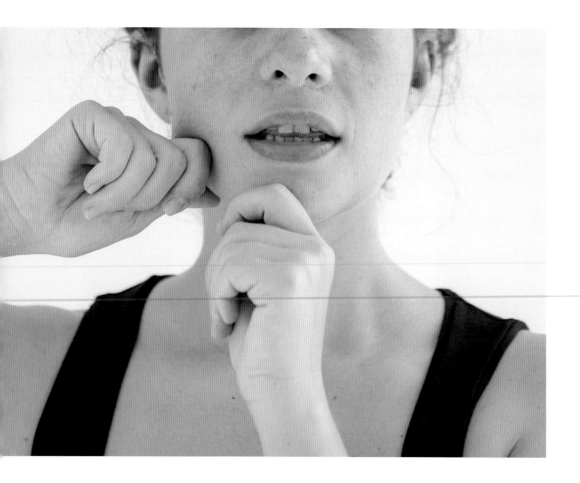

And yet, just as your body's muscles lose tone with age and underuse, so it is with the muscles in your face. Your facial muscles are directly attached to your skin, so when your muscle mass declines, unfortunately your complexion sags and hollows too. In the same way that gym workouts keep your body toned, a facial fitness programme can get your complexion in shape.

FACE EXERCISE BENEFITS

Toning and strengthening the muscles under your face creates a natural lift. Facial exercise also improves circulation to the skin, bringing more oxygen and nutrients – vital for a youthful, healthy glow. And working your facial muscles improves lymph flow, reducing puffiness. Beauty experts believe the results you get from facial exercise are far preferable to cosmetic treatments. A filler, for instance, can treat a deep line but will still leave your skin slack. And regular injections of Botox, which freezes muscles, can cause them to start wasting.

A facial fitness programme can get your complexion in shape.

So, what are you waiting for? Get a step ahead of the celebs and plump up your face the natural way!

Complete two sets of each of the exercises below once a day, for five days a week for best results. In addition, every day after applying an intensive moisturizer, use light pinching all over your face to get the blood flowing and to feed your skin cells with nutrients.

YOUR FACIAL WORKOUT

The following facial exercises have been devised by celebrity face guru Eve Fraser. Together, they work on all areas of your face.

BASIC
Stimulates all the facial muscles

- With your back teeth lightly together, touch your face very lightly with your index fingers just above the corners of your mouth. Your lips should part slightly as you lift.

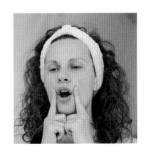

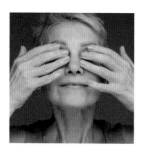

EYELIDS
Lifts your eyes
- Place the pads of three fingers firmly across both of your raised eyebrows. Hold your hands slightly diagonally outwards.
- Then, resting your fingers firmly on the browbone, blink six times.
- Next, working against the resistance of your fingers, try to close your eyelids in four slow downward moves. Hold this exercise for a count of 10.
- Relax for a few moments and repeat the exercise. But this time place the pads of your fingers on your eye socket bone without resting them on your eyelids.

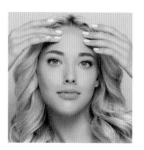

FOREHEAD
Targets frown lines
- Place your index fingers firmly along the length of your brows, which should be relaxed.
- Then, moving against the resistance of your fingers, lift your forehead muscles without raising your eyebrows. Hold for a count of 10.
- Finally, close your eyes and feel your forehead muscles slowly relaxing.

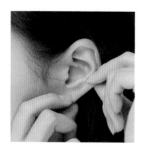

EARS
Stimulates flow of blood to facial muscles and skin
- With your index fingers and thumbs, hold the top rim of your ears and pull up. Using small rotations between your fingers and thumbs, massage the area.
- Move down all around the rim of the ears to the lobe, pulling your ears out gently and massaging them.
- Continue up to the top of your ear again. Repeat this for one minute.
- With your index fingers, make brisk circular movements over the surface of the ears and massage all its crevices and spirals with the pads of your index fingers.

FEED YOUR FACE

A nutritious diet doesn't just boost your health and reduce your risk of age-related disease – it can make you look more youthful too. Here's how to eat to boost your looks…

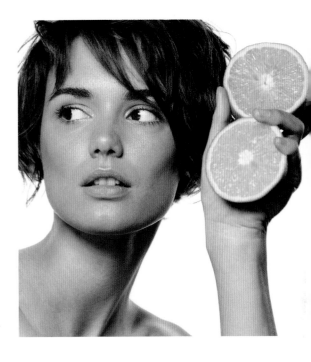

We've all been through periods in our lives when we haven't had the time or inclination to eat healthily. And you don't need us to tell you that it shows on your skin almost immediately. It stands to reason – the skin is your body's largest organ, it's constantly renewing itself and it's nutrient-hungry.

Now scientists are discovering more about the intricate relationship between complexion and diet. Many experts, including the world-renowned dermatologist Dr Nicholas Perricone, author of *The Wrinkle Cure*, believe the typical western diet is a major cause of wrinkles. In particular, Dr Perricone singles out our love of sugar and simple carbohydrates – white bread, for example – as a problem area. He argues that a sugary diet encourages collagen fibres (which should keep your skin springy and firm) to stiffen in a process known as glycation, leading to visible ageing.

Your skin relies on a nourishing supply of oxygen from your blood. So, as well as avoiding sugar, anything that compromises your circulation – in particular saturated and trans fats – are a big no-no. As are dehydrating tipples, such as alcohol and caffeine.

Conversely, research is showing that certain foods, such as antioxidant-rich fruit and vegetables and omega-3-rich oily fish, can boost skin by reducing inflammation (a key cause of ageing in our skin and body) and fighting free radicals.

Citrus fruits are a good source of dietary antioxidants – especially in the peel.

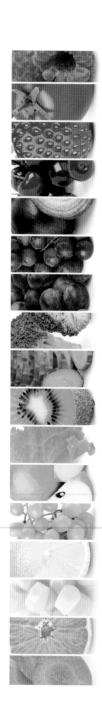

RECIPE FOR SKIN SUCCESS

A skin-boosting diet should include all the food groups (fats, carbs and protein), plenty of water and be replete in antioxidants to fight free-radical damage and boost your immune system.

BOOST YOUR COLLAGEN

It's important to feed your body with the nutrients it needs to produce and maintain its scaffolding tissue – in other words, protein and vitamin C. Eggs are great anti-agers; as well as being a great source of protein, they also contain the detoxifying amino acid cystine, which aids the formation of collagen. Vitamin B1 (thiamine) has also been shown to slow down the loss of collagen fibres, so increase your intake of vitamin B-rich wholegrains, including brown rice, and eat more oatmeal and sunflower seeds.

HYDRATE AND KEEP INFLAMMATION AT BAY

Two to three litres of water a day is a must – more if you're in hotter climes or exercising rigorously. In addition, essential fatty acids (EFAs) available in fish, nuts and seeds can help maintain your skin's hydration levels. There is some evidence that fish oil can help reduce sun damage, thinning of the skin and wrinkle formation. We know that EFAs have calming, anti-inflammatory qualities too, as do B vitamins, so stock up on wholemeal pasta, nuts and seeds, fish, chicken and avocados.

PROTECT YOUR CELLS

Antioxidants are foremost in your battle against ageing skin. A good antioxidant rule of thumb is to eat a rainbow of vividly coloured fresh fruit and vegetables. Dark green leafy veg, blood oranges, red grapes, carrots, squash and red (bell) peppers are all super-potent. Pack in berries, cherries and green tea, which all contain proanthocyanidins, which are antioxidants, plus green veg for free-radical scavenging carotenoids, and tomatoes and red fruits for lycopene, which helps reduce inflammation and protects the skin from UV damage.

A YOUTHFUL SMILE

There's nothing more ageing than yellowing teeth and receding gums, so time-proof your teeth now and stay looking younger for longer.

Given what we ask of them, our teeth are super-tough, but the natural ageing process takes its toll. And when it does, this can affect how youthful you look. When your gums recede and teeth darken and wear down, it can change the structure of your face, making you look older than you are. Gum problems can lead to tooth loss and even cardiovascular problems too, so looking after your oral health can really pay off.

STAINED REPUTATION

As you age, the enamel on your teeth becomes more translucent, and dentine (the layer beneath the enamel) naturally darkens. Add daily consumption of staining foodstuffs into the mix and discoloration starts to appear. A dazzling white Hollywood shine can look totally unnatural, but if you want to lighten the load on your teeth, try whitening toothpastes and speak to your dentist about professional treatments. It's best to avoid DIY home-whitening kits – research shows they can weaken your enamel. Instead, limit your intake of teeth-staining food and drinks (tea, coffee and red wine are the worst culprits), chew sugar-free gum after meals and always clean your teeth thoroughly.

TOP TEETH TIPS

Keeping your teeth youthful is all about common-sense habits.

- Clean and floss your teeth twice a day. Have check-ups and professional teeth cleaning every six months.
- When you're pregnant, your teeth and gums are more prone to problems – so good habits are important. You're allowed free NHS dental check-ups and treatment during pregnancy.
- Minimize acid erosion. Keep sugary foods, fizzy drinks, acidic fruits and juices to a minimum.
- After eating, sip on plain water and chew sugar-free gum to restore your mouth's natural pH level.
- Temper your alcohol intake. Not only can some drinks damage enamel, but excess drinking can increase your risk of developing mouth cancer.
- Calcium is vital for strong teeth, and omega 3 (in oily fish) is said to help dampen gum disease inflammation.
- If you think you have an allergy from amalgam or silver fillings, which may show as ulcerated patches on the skin or mouth, see your dentist or GP.

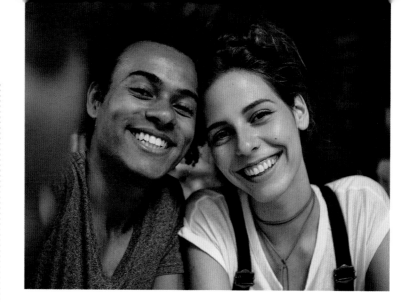

BYE GUM!

The risk of gum problems rises as you age, as accumulated bacteria grow in pockets at the root of your teeth, which can lead to infection and tooth loss. Practise good oral hygiene – floss and brush your teeth night and morning to remove plaque. Also, visit a hygienist twice a year for a 'deep clean'. Don't over-brush – gums naturally recede with age, and this can accelerate it. Visit your dentist if receding gums have left any metal crown root pins exposed.

THE DAILY GRIND

Many people unwittingly 'brux' or grind their teeth at night. This can be hereditary or triggered by stress, and can leave you with worn, extra-sensitive teeth. Your dentist should identify if you're a teeth-grinder and fit you with a night guard to prevent gnashing. Damage can be repaired with enamel veneers, but they're expensive and can be painful to have fitted.

DRY AND ARID

Hydration levels in your mouth plummet as you age. Because saliva works to neutralize acids, a dry mouth increases your risk of decay and gum problems. Chewing sugar-free gum after meals can help the problem and your dentist may recommend saliva-like mouthwashes.

HERE COMES THE SUN!

We all I feel better when the sun comes out, but as it's the leading cause of premature ageing, it's good to know how to protect yourself...

There are few things more uplifting than sunlight on your face, and a daily dose of sunshine is good for you – so much so that health bodies including Cancer Research UK and the National Osteoporosis Society recommend we enjoy 10 to 15 minutes in the sun, without sunscreen, daily in summer to safeguard our vitamin D levels.

However, there's a fine line between safe and unsafe exposure. Apart from not smoking, protecting your complexion from the sun is the most important thing you can do to prevent premature ageing. While ultraviolet B (UVB) rays cause burning by damaging your skin's DNA, it's the ultraviolet A (UVA) rays that are the main ageing enemies. They penetrate your skin and damage the structural fibres, which leads to photoageing – wrinkles and sagging. And prolonged exposure can increase your risk of skin cancer, one of the most common cancers in the UK. Experts say it takes just one episode of blistering sunburn before the age of 20 to double your chances of malignant melanoma in later life.

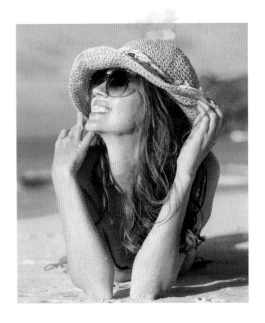

PREVENT AND PROTECT

After a series of high-profile campaigns, public awareness about sun damage is greater than ever, but many of us are still woefully lapse about healthy sun habits.

Sun protection isn't just for holidays abroad. Daily face protection is necessary, even in winter sun. Sunscreens are added to

Be sensible in the sun. Wear a wide-brimmed hat, sunglasses and protective clothing.

many skincare products, but don't burden your complexion with multiple shields, as they can irritate. Choose one product, such as a daily moisturizer or foundation, that provides broad-spectrum SPF 15 protection, so that it provides a barrier against both UVA and UVB rays.

In the UK, UVA protection is rated with a star system, varying from zero to five stars, so look for products with at least four stars. For more information visit www.sunsmart.org.uk.

Use a common-sense approach – if you spend the majority of your time outdoors, you'll need something stronger than an office worker would use. If you have sensitive skin, try products with natural mineral filters.

CHOOSE A HIGH FACTOR

If you're on your holidays or relaxing outdoors in the summer sun, apply a strong broad-spectrum sunscreen liberally to all exposed body parts. Cancer Research UK recommends at least SPF 15 with four stars or more, but the message is 'the higher the better'.

Apply generously and regularly. If you sweat a lot or enjoy water sports, apply protection more frequently. Don't forget to cover the forgotten or hard-to-reach parts, including your ears, lips and the backs of your legs. And check the expiry date on your sunscreen. Some creams will only last 12 months.

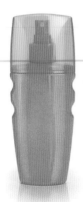

The sun's rays can be stronger at high altitudes, and the snow reflects them back at you, so cream up when skiing.

No sunscreen can provide 100 per cent protection, so be sensible about exposing yourself to the rays. Wear a wide-brimmed hat, sunglasses and protective clothing, and avoid sitting outdoors between 11 am and 3 pm. Take care even if you're driving or sitting in a conservatory – windows don't block UVA and UVB rays completely.

Sunbeds are not a safe alternative to sunbathing, and a fake tan won't protect you from sun damage – you'll still need to use sunscreen. And monitor your moles. Changes in size, shape or colour, bleeding and itching could be early signs of skin cancer.

MAKE-UP MASTERCLASS

Want to look 10 years younger? It's easier than you think!
The right products and techniques can take years off you.

You wouldn't necessarily want to wear the same clothes you did when
you were a teen, and the same principle applies to your make-up. Just as
your body shape alters and those hot pants may not be as appealing as
they once were, so too the changes to your skin require a fresh approach
to your make-up products. Today's cosmetics can work wonders – from
giving you dewy, fresh skin to concealing dark circles and blurring away
lines. With a few choice products and clever make-up tricks, you can
knock years off your face.

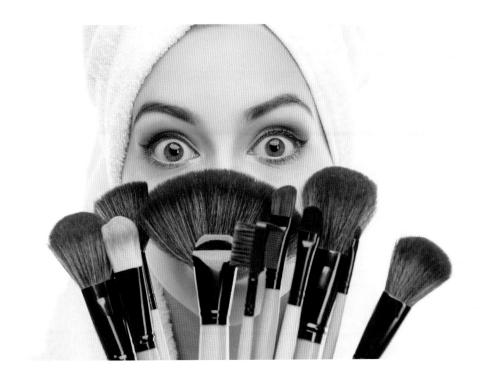

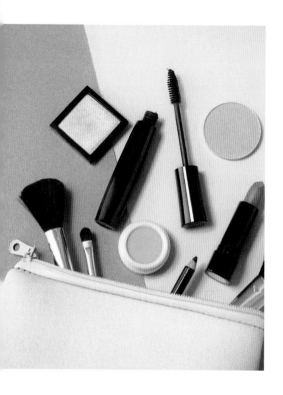

GIVE YOUR COSMETICS BAG A SPRING CLEAN

This is not simply to take years off your looks, but to protect your wellbeing too! A recent survey by the College of Optometrists found that 25 per cent of us use cosmetics that are more than four years old, putting us at risk of bacterial infections, including conjunctivitis. Experts recommend replacing mascara every six months and the main players – eyeshadow, lipstick and blusher – within two years.

GET A GLOW!

Dry, dull skin can make you look older. To recapture your youthful radiance, use a light-reflecting foundation – avoid flat matte – or a tinted moisturizer. Use a slightly damp brush to apply it and set with a fine and iridescent loose (not pressed) powder. Dab highlighter on your cheekbones, forehead and nose, and blend it in.

EVEN OUT YOUR SKIN TONE

Sun damage and hormonal changes can upset the evenness of your skin tone. Thankfully, there's an array of corrector and primer products to use after moisturizing and before layering on a light foundation. If you're suffering ruddy pigmentation, avoid red tones in your make-up, which will only draw attention to your problem.

BRIGHTEN YOUR EYES

Our eyes become smaller as we age. To brighten them, apply a light-reflecting concealer in the hollows under your eyes. Use a highlighter under your brows to add lift. If your eyelids are drooping, avoid blending deep shades into the sockets. Instead, start with a primer and then apply a neutral shade to lighten and even out your skin tone. Finish with eyeliner and mascara for definition.

THE EYEBROW FACELIFT!

Tweezing your eyebrows into shape is one of the easiest ways to add definition to your face. If you're not confident about plucking, get them done professionally – it's easy to keep the shape once you've been shown how.

- Invest in a good pair of slanted tweezers and pluck in a decent light.
- Hold a pencil vertically next to your nose and remove any hairs that fall inside the pencil line.

- To work out where your eyebrows end, move the pencil at a 45-degree angle from your nose tip, so it's diagonally across your face. Remove anything below the pencil.
- Now work on the shape of your brow by following its natural arch. Alternate which brow you pluck to get an even look.

NOTE: Thin brows are ageing, so make sure you don't overpluck.

MAKE LINES DISAPPEAR

Try one of the new magic line-smoother products. These generally include silicones and optical pigments that sit on the skin's surface and help blur the edges of your lines and wrinkles. Some products also include anti-ageing ingredients.

PLUMP UP YOUR CHEEKS

As we age, the youthful apples of our cheeks tend to slide downwards. Give your face an instant lift by applying a hint of blush onto your cheeks – the spot that plumps up when you smile. Opt for a cream blusher in a rose shade to recreate your natural youthful rosiness.

PUCKER UP!

Like every part of your body, your lips lose tone over time. You can add shape with a lip plumper containing hyaluronic acid. Outline with a neutral lip liner to add definition and prevent colour bleed. Shy away from matte lip colours, which can age you. Instead, opt for a light-reflective gloss to create the illusion of fullness. When you're outside in the sun, always apply an SPF lip balm.

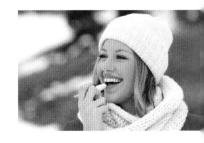

HOW TO HAVE PLUMP AND RADIANT SKIN

Want to plump up your skin without opting for fillers? Here are the key ingredients to look out for...

HYALURONIC ACID

This is a clear, viscous substance that your body produces naturally. It's found in greatest concentration in your skin, connective tissue and eyes. HA is like a sponge, holding up to a thousand times its weight in water, giving skin a soft, dewy and plump appearance.

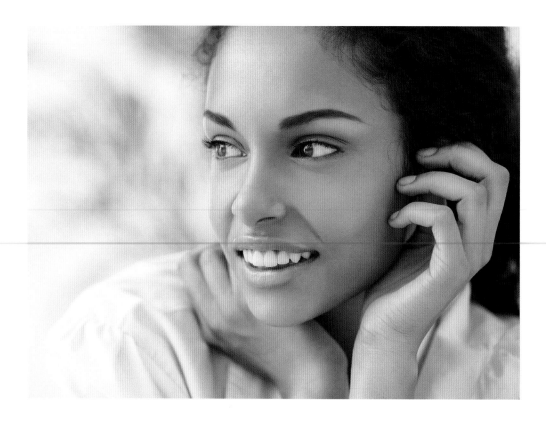

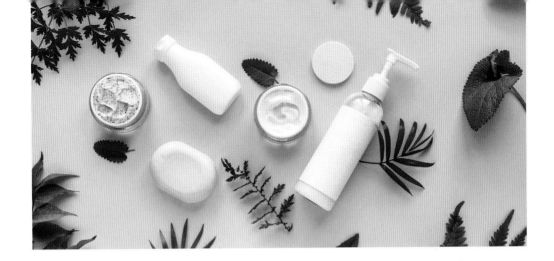

VITAMIN C

You need vitamin C to make collagen and keep skin healthy. It's a powerful antioxidant that helps protect skin from harmful free radicals (rogue molecules). Eating foods that are high in vitamin C will help to nourish your skin from the inside. Check for ascorbic acid (or L-ascorbic acid), as well as products that use pharmaceutical-grade vitamin C.

MEADOWFOAM

Meadowfoam oil is a lesser-known skincare secret, but one that is included in most menopausal skincare lines. Extracted from the flowers of the white meadowfoam plant (found in the US), the oil is rich in vitamins C and A, and other antioxidants.

RETINOL

Derived from vitamin A, retinol is added to skin products to boost collagen production, plump the skin, speed up skin renewal (sloughing off dead skin cells) and smooth fine lines and wrinkles.

COLLAGEN

Collagen is a protein made by the body. It's a major building block of skin, bones, muscles, tendons and ligaments. While there are skincare products that contain collagen, it's much more beneficial for the skin when taken as a supplement.

FABULOUS HAIR

Glossy, healthy hair is a sure way to make you feel amazing and get other people's heads turning. Here's how to keep yours at its youthful best...

We all know the difference a good – or bad – hair day can make to our mood and confidence. Healthy, conditioned locks, plus a good cut and colour are key to keeping you looking young.

Your hair is very much a barometer of your inner health and wellbeing. If you're run down, dieting or stressed, it won't be long before it shows up in your hair. Likewise, the good news is that if you eat well, exercise, de-stress and get plenty of sleep, you'll soon see an improvement in your hair. Treat your hair well from the outside too.

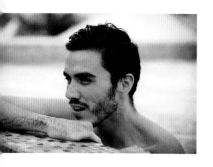

Overprocessing, whether with chemical treatments such as tinting and bleaching, heat treatments such as straighteners and tongs, or overexposure to sun and chlorine can all take a toll.

Your hair is made from the protein keratin, and is moisturized by your hair's oil – sebum – released from hair follicles in the scalp. Each hair is made up of overlapping layers of keratin. When the layers lie flat and smooth, your hair reflects the light, making it shine. When the layers are damaged, your hair is left looking dull and lifeless.

THINNING HAIR

Hair production gradually slows down as we age, so our hair naturally thins and dries. However, follicle foibles can strike at any age and, in total, it's estimated that 8 million British women are affected by some form of hair loss. Iron deficiency, pregnancy, some medications, autoimmune disease, episodes of stress or hormonal problems connected to the thyroid gland can trigger patches of baldness (alopecia) or overall shedding (telogen effluvium). Smoking can cause premature greying and thinning because it starves your follicles of youth-enhancing nutrients and oxygen. According to a study published in the *British Medical Journal*, smokers are four times more likely to have grey hair and increased hair loss. Excess alcohol is dehydrating and can deplete levels of iron in your body. And stress can also trigger major hair loss. See your GP if you're concerned about the health of your hair.

ANATOMY OF GREY

If we were to ask you to name the key signs of ageing, we'd wager grey hair would be up there. Like your skin, your hair gets its natural colour from a pigment called melanin, and as we age the cells that produce it, called melanocytes, gradually slow. *Et voilà*, grey hair!

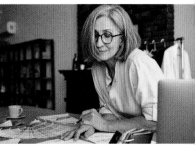

Exactly when you go grey – and it's a gradual process – is very much determined by your genes. A recent Danish twin study showed that while hair-thinning on the top of the head in women is partly connected to environmental and lifestyle factors, greying is largely beyond our control. That said, smoking and stress can accelerate it. Research done at Kanazawa University in Japan found that protracted levels of anxiety can damage the stem cells which help supply new melanocytes.

While some may find their first grey hair in their 20s, greying usually starts in our 30s and 40s. No hair colour is out-and-out more prone to greyness, but it shows up earlier on dark hair.

KEEP YOUR HAIR LOOKING YOUTHFUL
Soften up

A blunt, stiff or severe style can add years to your face, by drawing your eyes and cheeks down, so ask your hairstylist for some tousled layers to give your hair volume and your cheekbones definition. Have the best cut you can afford – a good hair style can make you look 10 years younger and fill you with confidence. Whether a maturing woman can carry off long hair is a great source of contention, but to be honest, you can carry off whatever style you want, provided you look after it. Irrespective of the length of your mane, keep updating it and take indulgently good care of it.

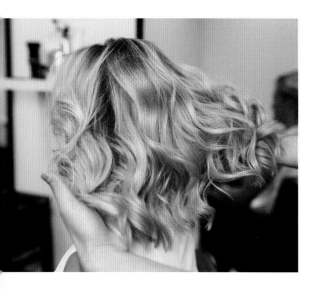

Colour sense

Remember all the guidelines we gave you about your make-up colours? They're relevant to your hair too. Cover up grey, yes, but avoid harsh dye jobs, matte and unnatural shades. Go for soft colours that flatter your complexion – that means shades that are only a couple of shades from lighter or darker than your natural hair colour. Ideally, have your hair professionally coloured at a salon at least once to get advice on the best shade for your skin tone.

There are some ultra-sophisticated techniques on the market – modern colourants are multi-toned and contain illuminating pigments that can transform ageing hair. Maximize your colour with colour-extending products which contain UV protectors and are designed to seal the hair cuticle.

Add volume

Get your hair tended to regularly – the longer and more unkempt it is, the less bounce and swing it will have. For added oomph and depth, ask your stylist for a layered style. Try using big Velcro or heated rollers and techniques such as backcombing. And add some volumizing products into your hair care regime.

Moisture must-haves

As well as thinning, your hair gets drier over the years as oil production slows. Keep your hair glossy by avoiding straighteners and other scorching hot appliances and dehydrating treatments, such as bleaching and perming. Protect your hair from chlorine by wearing a cap when you swim. Use replenishing intensive treatments and shine sprays regularly to bring back shine and make your hair more manageable. Naturalbased products may help, as they don't contain moisture-stripping detergents.

Feed your hair

A chronic deficiency of iron, B vitamins and zinc can exacerbate hair loss, so make sure you're eating a wide and balanced diet. Your hair is made from protein, so this is the most important food group for it. Essential fatty acids, present in nuts, seeds (or their oils) and oily fish, will help boost its condition. Add seaweeds such as arame, nori and wakame to your diet – use them in soups and stir fries, as they're rich in hair-friendly nutrients such as iodine, folate and magnesium. Consider a hair supplement if you need an extra boost.

UV protection

Your hair and scalp are as susceptible to sun damage as the rest of your body. Over-exposing your hair to the sun can damage the molecular structure, so it can become brittle, dry and dull. For protection, wear a hat or scarf and apply UV barrier sprays when you're out in sun.

Go with the flow

Good circulation to the scalp ensures your hair gets the oxygen and nutrients it needs to flourish. Regular aerobic exercise gives your circulation a kick-start and reduces stress, so this is a must for healthy hair. A regular home scalp massage is a good idea: using oil, move your fingers over your scalp and neck in small, but firm circular movements. Leave the oil in for 30 minutes, then shampoo and condition.

Soothe sensitivity

Just as the skin on your body becomes drier and therefore more sensitive as you age, so does your scalp. Avoid chemical-laden products, heat treatments and abrasive dyes to help alleviate mild itching and flaking, and try soothing scalp lotions or dandruff-relief shampoos.

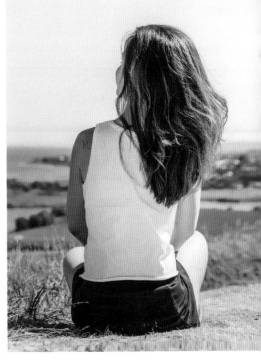

CONTRIBUTORS

Antonia Kanczula

Eve Boggenpoel

Lyndon Gee

Natalie Millman

Ladan Soltani

Charlotte Vöhtz

Jennifer Irvine